From Parent to Child about Sex

From Parent to Child about Sex

Including Questions for Discussion and Thought

by

WILSON W. GRANT, M.D.

ZONDERVAN PUBLISHING HOUSE
A DIVISION OF THE ZONDERVAN CORPORATION
GRAND RAPIDS, MICHIGAN

Contents

Contents

PART FIVE
WHEN PARENTS NEED HELP

From Parent to Child about Sex

PART ONE

◆

BIRDS, BEES, STORKS
AND OTHER MYTHS

Chapter 1

Introduction: Sex!

Sex!

No other word in the English language is so powerful.

The very sound of the word "sex" is enough to turn many pink with embarrassment. To others, it stimulates flights of fantasy; for some it brings about wishful thinking or pleasant memories. To all of us, sex is an extremely important part of life. But to all too many of us, sex and the feelings surrounding it are too little understood.

The definition of sex can be as narrow or as broad as one would want to make it. While in the most simple form it means "the condition of being male or female," others would give sex a broader meaning, calling it the elemental force or drive that promotes life and leads one to develop his or her unique personality as a man or a woman. Others, including an apparent majority of our culture, vulgarize the word sex to mean simply, "sex appeal"; "sex appetite" or "intercourse."

It is the broader meaning of sex with which we will be dealing in this book. Thus when we speak of sex, we mean everything in any way connected with our feelings of masculinity or femininity, or with female-male relationships.

We educate our children about finance and space flight; we teach them to read poetry and play volleyball; but all too often we as parents, churches and schools are silent about sex. Certainly this intense and complex aspect of a child's life deserves attention. Children, including preschoolers and maturing adolescents, are desperately searching for answers to their questions about sex. Sexuality does not just suddenly spring into being at puberty, or as some would believe, at marriage. Rather it influences the development of the individual through each of life's stages.

Thus the need for sex education is real. True, a parent's attitude toward sex (i.e., that it is nasty, that it is proper, or that it is nothing worth protesting about) is often fixed. Yet I believe there are many Christian parents who are searching for a way to convey the proper attitudes and information about sex to their children but do not know how. That is the reason for this book.

Most materials dealing with sex education take the plumbing approach — emphasizing the physical and anatomical aspect of sexual development. This book tries to look at sexuality as a whole. While not ignoring the plumbing, it is intended to help parents, particularly Christian parents, understand the more complex and important aspect of sex education — that of attitude and philosophy. The moral issues will be dealt with frankly. Practical ways of dealing with sexuality at each stage of the child's development will be discussed.

Actually the easiest part of sex education is teaching the facts such as reproductive biology. After all, these are just facts and can be looked up in books, or the child can be given a book to read by himself. But the most demanding need of growing youth is to know what the facts mean and how to handle the emotions raised by the facts. This is where morality and social customs come in, and this is where most parents as well as youth become confused.

Actually, we cannot separate morality from the factual aspect of sexuality.

A group of adolescent boys were being instructed in the anatomy of the sex organs. Eventually, the subject of sexual intercourse came up. Soon from the back of the room a timid question was heard. "Is it wrong to have sexual intercourse before marriage?"

Such a question is more the usual than the exception. Certainly teenagers are interested in the facts, but they also want to know what to do with these facts.

To such a question by a teenager we might respond, "I am not concerned about the morals of the case, therefore I can't answer." But by doing this we are giving a moral opinion. For we are saying that "the subject is not important enough for me to have an opinion," or that "morals are not related to the facts of sexual intercourse." And either of these statements is a moral judgment.

On the other hand it is an error to propound a code of do's and don't's to youth while not giving them an explanation for the rules or not helping them to understand the facts of their bodies and emotions. This is sometimes the approach of parents and churches and, more often than not, it leaves the young people confused and at the mercy of emotions and drives they do not understand.

This is not a book of rules and regulations. It seeks to give parents information about how children learn, grow, and think; to help parents formulate their own attitude toward sex; and to help them feel free to communicate with their children.

Questions For Discussion and Thought

1. What mental image do you have when you think of the word "sex"?
2. What definition of sex did you learn from your parents?
3. Are you satisfied with the sex education you received from your parents?
4. Are you satisfied with the sex education you have given your children up to this point?

Chapter 2

From Back Seats to Bathroom Walls

Jane hesitated. Worry clouded her fifteen-year-old face as she stepped into the office. The physician, a family friend, motioned for her to sit down.

"Now tell me what's bothering you," he invited.

"I'm confused and worried," Jane began timidly. "You see, my parents haven't told me very much about sex. Mother has always said that nice people don't talk about it. She even hides the newspaper when there is something about sex in it."

Jane paused, her eyes fixed on a worn spot in the rug.

"Doctor, my real question is this," she blurted out, "Can a girl get pregnant if she keeps her clothes on?"

Fortunately Jane was not pregnant. But she needed help desperately and her plight tells us many things about children and sex. Some parents believe that sex is a subject to be talked about as little as possible; most are plainly embarrassed and uncomfortable talking about it; a few openly oppose sex education thinking that information about sex will corrupt their children. Jane points out the fallacy of these philosophies.

The question is not whether our children will get a sex education — they will get it. The real question is *what kind* of sex education they will get and *where* they will get it.

If they do not learn about this vital subject at home from their parents or from other responsible adults, they will learn about it elsewhere. Thousands of young girls, like Jane, are learning about sexual intercourse in the back seats of automobiles because they have not learned about it from their parents. They are easily overrun by emotions that they are not able to control because they have never felt free to talk with an adult about them.

Many preadolescent boys learn male and female anatomy from drawings on bathroom walls because the real names of body parts have never been discussed with them. A few moments spent scanning the latest art work over the public toilet bowl leaves no doubt about the poor quality of such an education.

Parents who think they can shield their children from "sex" simply by not talking about it should stop for a moment and look at the drive-in movie ads in the daily newspaper, or glance at the magazines available in their own home for the teenagers to read, or simply notice what is splashed on the TV in living color. Information, more commonly, misinformation, runs rampant throughout our society.

Yes, the real question is not whether our children will receive a sex education, but what kind. Sad as it is, Jane's problem is all too common. Her mother can hide the newspaper or refuse to talk about sex, but she can be sure that Jane and others like her will listen to friends and experiment.

A poll of 1,000 teenagers revealed that sex information was gained in the following ways:

- only 32 percent of the girls and 15 percent of the boys were informed about sex by their parents;
- 53 percent of the boys and 42 percent of the girls found out from friends of their own age;
- 15 percent pieced together the information they had received from other sources;
- 56 percent of these young people acquired their sex knowledge between the sixth and ninth grades

and 18 percent learned about sex before the fifth grade;

- a full 88 percent of these young people felt they needed more information about sex than they had received from their parents.

(As quoted in the March 1962 issue of the *Journal of Health — Physical Education — Recreation.*)

School age children and youth today have acquired much sex education. Their peers and mass media have filled them with images and suggestive fantasies that distort the real meaning of sex. Advertising insists that its products give sex allure which alone makes one attractive; marriage is shown as simply playing house with the latest gadgets. Aroused with curiosity, children may try to get answers from their parents. But too often they find us, their parents, too busy, embarrassed, or misinformed, or they just don't find us at all. So their answers must come from elsewhere.

Jane teaches us something else about sex education. What young people don't know about sex is hurting them, and hurting them badly. Children who don't find answers to their questions, spoken or unspoken, concerning sex, will turn to their peers. Often stimulated by curiosity, they begin to experiment. This experimentation can have dire effects. It may lead to pregnancy with its resulting physical and psychological problems; it often leads to early and poorly planned marriages; it almost always produces guilt that interferes with the young person's future adjustment.

Over the past twenty years there has been a marked increase in teenage marriages. This is alarming because of the disastrous outcome of many such marriages. The United States Census Bureau shows that the divorce rate in teenage marriages is three times as high as in marriages where the partners are between the ages twenty-one to twenty-five. In one study, three out of four teenage marriages eventually broke up. These marriages not only tend to shorten the education and job preparation of the youth, but they also affect the next generation: teenage parents produce a higher percentage of premature babies, and more of their babies are born ill due to lack of prenatal care.

Pregnancy in unmarried teenagers is a disaster for everyone involved. Some of the pregnancies result in illegal abortion with the attending dangers to the life of the girl. In most cases, the young mother gives up the child for adoption; occasionally she decides to keep the baby in spite of the many problems involved. Whatever the outcome, all of these pregnancies result in sadness and heartbreak, not only for the girl and boy involved, but for their families and for the infant. The young parents often fail to complete their education. When they marry, they more often than not end up divorced. They often become trapped in a self-destructive cycle consisting of failure to continue their education, dependence on others for support, failure to establish a stable family life, and repeated pregnancies.

Also young people are being hurt by venereal disease because of their lack of information. Both syphilis and gonorrhea can now be successfully cured. In spite of this, we are in the midst of a spiraling epidemic of these two diseases. Most of the new cases are among teenagers. Dr. Celia Deschin made a study of 600 teenagers who came to a venereal disease clinic in New York City. It was learned that only 21 percent of them had received any sex information from their parents. Only 10 percent of these young people had an adequate knowledge of the disease for which they were being treated.

What young people don't know about sex is hurting them! It is ironical that we educate our children so much about the world in which they will make a living but teach them so little about living. In so many ways, we glorify marriage, family life, motherhood, and fatherhood, but we leave the preparation for these responsibilities largely to chance.

A Sunday school class of thirteen-year-old girls was discussing some of their sexual questions. The girls were embarrassed to say the word, "intercourse," but referred to the act as "doing it." Of course the embarrassment and mystery with which adults treat such words only increases the adolescent's curiosity and makes even the saying of the word itself sexually stimulating. Sometimes even educated parents instruct their children not to use proper sexual terms. One girl was told by her mother that saying the word "pregnant" was naughty. She was twelve years old before she learned that you could not become pregnant by holding hands, kissing, or by just saying "pregnant."

Not all children receiving inadequate sex education at home are from poor families or broken homes. Many are from middle class, educated families and many are from families who are regular church attenders. Alice was one of a group of thirteen-year-olds attending a discussion on sex at her church. Her father was an executive and the family lived in the "good" part of town. The question of "the navel" came up and Alice asked, "What's the belly button for?" When asked what she thought it was for, she replied that it was made by a big needle the doctor used to feed the baby after it was born. When asked where she got this information, she said that one of her friends had told her.

The child who is faced with the withholding or the distorting of sex information by his parents perceives one of two things: Sex is either unimportant (which he can hardly believe because of the intensity of his own feelings); or sex is bad (which again is hard to believe since sex plays such an important part in the life of humanity).

Thus we as parents, (yes, and as Christian parents), are to often shortchanging our children when it comes to sex. Our children are caught up by this fundamental force of life, yet we give them so little aid or understanding to help them cope with the forces that are bursting within them. Too often we don't even admit that these forces exist. Thus our children have no choice but to look elsewhere — and that elsewhere is completely inadequate.

There are several reasons for this but a prominent one is that in our society, too many parents look on sex as dirty and a subject not to be talked about. When it is talked about, it is in a threatening way. One mother remarked that her main objective in sex education was to create enough fear in the mind of her daughter so that she would not become pregnant.

"Fear is a poor way to prevent pregnancy," I answered. "If your only goal is to prevent pregnancy, why not give your daughter contraceptives? Then you can sit back and relax."

This mother was shocked by my suggestion. Personally I do not believe in giving contraceptives to young unmarried girls. But contraceptives would probably be more healthy for her daughter than the misinformation and fear that the mother was implanting in her and they certainly would do a better job of preventing pregnancy. It has been shown that most of the girls who become pregnant out of wedlock come from homes where sex information was either distorted or sparse.

To a few parents the main goal in sex education may be only to head off such problems as venereal disease and pregnancy. But I think most parents honestly want to give their children more information. To be sure, none of us want our daughters getting pregnant or any of our children having premature sexual experiences. The best way to reach that goal, however, is not a negative, but a positive approach about sexuality.

A child's interest in sexual subjects is innate and God-given. It cannot be shut up. Honest sex education which helps the child see sex in perspective and from an early age helps him learn how to control his sexual feelings will be much more successful in preventing premature sexual experience than harsh warnings, threats, or ignorance.

But the Christian parent's goal is even greater than this. Our goal should be to help our children understand that sex is one of God's greatest gifts. Our goal should be to help our children develop a capacity for mature love, and help them become a *responsible* and *responsive* man or woman.

Before we can successfully discuss "how" to teach children about sex, we must decide "what" to teach. For it is the value system and attitudes of his parents that will ultimately determine a child's attitudes and actions about sex. Thus the next two chapters will concern themselves with concepts of sexuality and the meaning of sex.

Questions For Discussion and Thought

1. Where did you learn most of your information about sex while growing up?
2. As a child did you get the idea that sex was basically good or bad?
3. How old were you when you learned the truth about where babies came from?
4. Would you want your child to learn this fact in the same way?
5. As a child what were some of the misconceptions you had about where babies came from?
6. What is the goal of a real Christian sex education?

PART TWO

◆

CHRISTIAN MORALITY! NEW MORALITY! NO MORALITY!

Chapter 3

Sex Is Love? Love Is Sex? Sex Is Sin?

One reason why we parents, particularly Christian parents, have been uncomfortable in relaying sexual information to our children is that we are unsure of what we think, or should think, about sex. We are pulled one way by those who proclaim that sexual expression with or without love does more good than harm. On the other hand we are influenced by those who label all aspects of sex a necessary evil and any expression of sex shameful. Torn between the hangups of the Victorian and Puritan past and the "free love" scene of today, we don't quite know how to feel about sex, much less what to say about it. We see that sexual feelings and drives are not all bad, but we are still unsure what will happen if these feelings are talked about openly.

Today we frequently hear that "sex is nothing to be ashamed of." In one sense that is certainly true. One of the major themes of this book is that we should not be ashamed of the fact that the human race reproduces itself in a certain way or that the experiencing of sex gives pleasure. But we certainly should be ashamed of the state to which man's sexuality and use, or accurately misuse of sex, has fallen. So often man has distorted the true purpose of sex to where in the end it brings pain rather than pleasure.

Distortions of sex and its meaning run rampant in our society today. Let us first look at some of these, then we will take a hard look at what the Bible has to say about sex.

DISTORTIONS OF SEXUALITY

Sex Is Sin!

"The reason I started to drink," Mary Smith remarked, "was guilt about my sexual feelings. As a small child I was taught that anything connected with sex was evil — that God hated sex. From my mother I got the impression that it was sinful to have any sexual feelings. At college I found myself around other young people of both sexes and I no longer could deny that I was a sexual person. Even though I married a young man I loved, I was so inhibited about sex that we never had a happy marriage or satisfactory sex life. I began to drink in an attempt to bury my feelings."

After a long period of therapy, Mary was able to overcome her guilt about sex. She is now happy in her marriage relationship, but the scars of her unhappy past cannot be erased. Such inhibitions about sex are all too common — too many people have a sneaking suspicion that sex is always dirty. Although only a small percentage of these individuals may be driven to drink, thousands are not able to experience peace and happiness in marriage because they have unnatural guilt about sex. Husbands and wives who were taught as children that sex equals sin often suffer such unfortunate sequelae as pain, frigidity, impotency, and premature ejaculation. These sequelae may persist long after the marriage ceremony is over, even if the couple is no longer conscious of their guilt and fervently desire sexual happiness.

Repression of sexuality characterized the Victorian world of our grandparents and lingers to a great extent in our own. We have invented scores of euphemisms to describe — or attempt to hide — the body functions. We speak of chamber pots and water closets, of "pee pee" instead of urinate, of "doing it" instead of intercourse; one is not pregnant, but "in a family way." Although sex is something people may "do," they are not supposed to enjoy it.

Men and women who think sex is basically evil often try to deny their own sexual feelings and push them out of their consciousness. The flaw in this plan is that sexual feelings are such a basic part of human makeup that one cannot deny them for long. The sex drives lie smoldering in the subconscious waiting for an unguarded moment to pop out. They often reappear in disguised form such as anxiety, nervousness and physical illness.

June grew up in a family where any mention of sex was taboo. She was never told anything about menstruation but picked up ideas from other girls, some not too well informed. When she was twelve years old she asked her mother how babies were born.

"Don't talk about that," her mother replied. "That's shameful."

During adolescence, June felt the same attraction for boys that other girls felt. But she repressed these thoughts and spent all her time studying. When asked for a date she found excuses not to go. She secretly wanted to accept, but she was afraid of impulses that she could not deny, yet did not want to admit. Her sexual energy was channeled into her work. She was an honor student and later on an excellent fourth grade teacher. But she gradually became a caustic, bitter spinster who resented the fact that life was passing her by. June, like many who grow up believing that sex and sexual feelings are all evil, became severely crippled emotionally.

Such repression and suspicion of sex has been all too common in the past. Realizing the great power of sexual drives and that they were often used for pain and destruction, some Christians have mistakenly chosen to bury their sexuality. To do this they have labeled all things sexual evil and tried to blot sex from their life. Thus virginity and celibacy have been glorified in times past as a greater good than marriage itself.

Sex Is Love!

We hear much today about the sexual revolution and its ethics of "new morality." This new morality represents another distortion of sexuality that in one sense is an overreaction to the previous concept that sex is always sin.

Although the modern sexual revolution means different things to different people, one thing it does mean is that many young people are discovering that sex is not evil or ugly. But after making this discovery they don't know what to do with it. Often young people, in rebelling against our society's confusion about sex, rebound to the new morality which in essence proclaims that there are no hard and fast rules governing sexual expression. Whether an act is moral depends on the circumstances at the time and on how the people involved "feel."

To many young people sex becomes simply a way of expressing their affection for another person. One sixteen-year-old high school girl put it this way. "Johnny's a nice guy. Why shouldn't I give him what he wanted? Sure we made love." Many college students demand their "right" to have sexual intercourse whenever they wish in their college dorms or elsewhere. The new morality proclaims that sex with love is permissible as long as a boy or girl does not fall "in love" with two people at the same time.

Under these circumstances sexual relationships become transient affairs involving little responsibility. "To make love" is equated with sexual intercourse. In fact the new morality breaks down at this point — its concept of love. It fails to distinguish between superficial love that says, "I love sex and want you" (as a sexual partner); or true romantic love that seeks to honor the one loved and says, "She's the only girl for me." When one really loves a person, he or she does not want to use that person to satisfy his own desires but wants to commit himself or herself to the lover. That commitment is, in essence, the foundation of marriage. Real love, then, means much more than "to make love," or feel sexually attracted to another person.

Sex as God!

Deifying sex is another distortion of the true meaning of sex that is all too common in our society. To many moderns, sex is a god. The seeking of sexual expression is an obsession that ocupies most of their time and effort. Constant energy is pumped into efforts to make themselves more attractive to the opposite sex. Their conversation constantly turns to sex in the form of jokes, bragging of sexual prowess, or seduction.

Such behavior reminds us of the ancient pagans who built temples to their sexual gods and goddesses and used both male and female prostitution as a part of their "worship." It was this distortion of sex that the God of the Hebrews warned them against when they began to mix with the worshipers of Baal who inhabited Palestine. To this day, one can see among the ruins baking under the Middle Eastern sun statues of Astarte, goddess of fertility, with her exquisitely carved genitals exposed. Much of the Greek and Roman world worshiped Venus, goddess of love. Even today her name is often equated with love itself. In her temples sex was supreme and wild abandon to sexual urges the norm.

The modern pagans do not call themselves religious, but they are just as preoccupied with sex as the ancients were. In this sense, sex is god to many in our society today. In fact, a Martian visiting earth would probably return home to report that sex was the American god.

Sex Is Fun!

Treating sex as just a plaything or another form of entertainment — a pastime — is a prevalent distortion of the true worth of sex. *Playboy* Magazine, the chief exponent of this philosophy, boasts that the magazine "naturally includes sex as one of the ingredients in its total entertainment package for the young urban male." This is exactly what the hedonistic philosophy does to women: it turns them into big bosomed, leggy packages of entertainment. They are not persons or individuals, but stereotyped packages of "frisky fun."

This philosophy turns a woman into one of the expendable consumer items available to the "sophisticated male" who then brags about the number of packages he has untied. Sex is a commodity to be bought and sold on the open market. A girl's value is measured only in terms of a big bosom, curvaceous figure, and pretty legs. The ultimate manifestation of sex is the orgasm — not the human relationships associated with it.

In reality this hedonistic concept of sex is a very superficial one and often represents a person's effort to escape the deeper relationships and commitments that are present in real love and true sexuality.

Each one of these distortions of sex is bankrupt in its own way. Whether a college student expressing his individuality, or a sex saturated individual bowing at the throne of sex, or a "young urban male" searching for a sexual binge, the individuals involved are prostituting the real meaning of sex and short changing themselves.

While sex is an expression of love, love is much more than sex; while sex should be fun, it is not a toy; and while one's sexual feelings are very important in the development of the personality, sex is not the most important thing in life.

The Bible and Sex

The Bible is a very sexual book!

This fact may surprise many Christians and shock some, but it is true. The Bible speaks without embarrassment or shame about sex.

We need not read far into Genesis before we discover that man, by creation, is a psychophysical being. The Bible does not divide man into a separate soul and body, but views man as spirit, mind, and body all welded together into one being. As the Bible focuses on man's spiritual pilgrimage, it does not ignore man's physical nature. Sex, because it is an important aspect of our lives, is dealt with frankly.

The creation story itself, suggests that man's sexual nature serves two purposes:

The most obvious function is that of procreation. "So God created man in his own image, in the image of God created he him; male and female created he them. And God blessed them, and God said unto them, 'Be fruitful and multiply, and replenish the earth . . .'" (Gen. 1: 27, 28). All societies and cultures have recognized this aspect of man's sexuality. Even the most confirmed Victorians admit that sex is necessary for reproduction, even though some act as if it is a necessary evil.

A less obvious, but just as important, function of sex is unification. "And the Lord God said, it is not good that man should be alone; I will make a helpmate for him" (Gen. 2:18). God made man and woman in such a way that each is incomplete without the other. In a way they are like a key and a lock; they are made to fit together — apart they do not completely fulfill their

God ordained purpose. In the relationship of marriage, a man and woman together unlock the beauty and meaning of sex and life itself.

The Old Testament speaks openly of sexual matters and is not embarrassed by them. First of all, it knows none of our modern uneasiness in talking about sex. Normal sexual relationships are not ignored. Over and over the Bible states that a man ". . . knew his wife and she conceived." This verb "to know" in the original language means "to have intercourse" and is translated as such by the newer versions of the Scriptures.

The Law of Moses forbade sexual intercourse by women only during the period of menstruation and childbirth and married men were ordered to abstain from intercourse only for religious reasons, thus implying that sexual relations were natural and good. Further, the Old Testament openly discusses the sexual sins of the individuals it chronicles. The escapades of Lot, the treachery of David and Bathsheba, and the prostitution of Hosea's wife are openly recorded.

One of the most unusual books in the Bible is the Song of Songs. This book stands among the most romantic literature ever written. Much of the book is a mystery, but in essence it appears to be a drama of two lovers raptly in love with each other. Their poetic dialogue is uninhibitedly recorded. For example, the bridegroom says to his lover, "Your navel is a rounded goblet that never shall want for spiced wine. Your belly is a heap of wheat fenced in by lilies. Your two breasts are like two fawns, twin fawns of a gazelle" (Chapter 7: 2, 3, N.E.B.). The bride replies, "I am my beloved's, his longing is all for me. Come, my beloved, let us go out into the fields to lie among the henna-bushes" (Chapter 7:10, 11, N.E.B.).

The exclusive oneness dramatized by these lovers is romantic love as it is meant to be experienced. It is obvious that to them sexual love is more than just a means of procreation. Some say that this book is an allegory of God's concern for Israel, others say that it is prophetic of Christ's love for the Church. In any case, it is significant that the sexual discovery of this couple is chosen to express God's concern and love for people. The most intimate relationship of man and woman is a shadow of God's love for all people. Certainly, it appears that God puts His seal of approval on sexual relationships by using this illustration to allegorize His relationship to people.

The New Testament, although not preoccupied with sex, acknowledges and approves of it. It is noteworthy that Jesus' first miracle was performed at a wedding and He apparently enjoyed the happiness of that occasion. Jesus spoke frankly on several occasions of the dangers in misusing sex. He spoke against sexual intercourse outside the bounds of marriage. Yet, He did not consider sexual sins as being any greater than other sins and He forgave prostitutes just as He forgave hypocrites and extortioners. The story of the woman taken in adultery shows the great compassion Jesus had for those who committed sexual sins. "Whomever among you is without sin cast the first stone" rings loud and clear through the ages.

The writer of Hebrews speaks just about as bluntly as one can about sex: "Marriage is honorable in all, and the bed undefiled" (Heb. 13:4). Can you find any more explicit approval for sex than that?

Thus the Bible treats sex honestly and frankly. It is not preoccupied with sex, but neither is it ashamed of it. Man is a whole being and cannot be cut up into bits and pieces. The Bible deals with the whole man and this includes his sexual nature.

The Bible has a positive attitude toward sex. As part of God's creation, sex is basically good. But like the rest of creation, it can be distorted into evil by imperfect creatures. The sex drive is a powerful force for good or evil depending on how men and women choose to express it. Realizing this, God sets down certain guidelines for the expression of human sexuality. In the next chapter, we will see how the Bible's concept of sex should influence our and our children's sexual behavior in the twentieth century.

Questions For Discussion and Thought

1. Are the attitudes about sex which you express in public the same as those you honestly feel?
2. Which distortion of sexuality was most prevalent when you were growing up?
3. Which distortion of sexuality is most prevalent in your community today?
4. Which distortion of sexuality is most misleading to young people?
5. How can we best convey to our children a wholesome Biblical concept of sex?

Chapter 4

◆

Guidelines for Sexual Expression

Responsibility

A young couple may treat sex casually and engage in sexual relations freely, but they can be assured that sex will not treat them casually. It is a fact, propounded in the Bible and rediscovered by modern science, that sexual actions produce consequences. Sexual feelings are among the most intense of man's emotions. This intensity dictates that sex not be taken lightly. To do so invites disaster.

The tragedy of David and Bathsheba is but one glaring example of the disastrous consequences which await those who misuse sex. Bathsheba, the beautiful wife of Uriah, one of David's top generals, caught the eye of the young king. Soon David and Bathsheba acted on their impulses and were having an intense affair. Eventually Bathsheba became pregnant. By this time, David and Bathsheba were caught in a web of murder, heartbreak and family tragedy from which they could not escape. From the ashes of their affair, a cruel web of sadness and pain was weaved. Later David repented of his misdeeds, but history could not be changed nor the scars erased.

David's prayer of repentance is one of the most poignant of all time: "Wash me thoroughly from mine iniquity, and cleanse me from my sin. For I acknowledge my transgressions; and my sin is ever before me"

(Ps. 51:2, 3). David and Bathsheba discovered the hard way that, indeed, sexual responsibility cannot be taken lightly.

A natural result of sexual intercourse is children with the awesome responsibility of parenthood. This in itself is reason enough to make sexual relationships a matter of serious judgment. Every time I visit an unmarried teenage girl in the labor and delivery room, I am impressed that the Bible's warning about the responsibility inherent in sexual actions is not passé. The fear, the anxiety, the regret that grips these girls between labor pains is convincing.

But some say, "Ah, but isn't some of the responsibility removed from sexual relationships in these days of effective birth control and liberal abortion laws?"

Even with the prospect of pregnancy erased, sex cannot be taken as casually as some would like. The emotional consequences can be just as devastating as the physical ones. Sexual intercourse is a physical commitment and, as such, it is a symbol of the emotional and spiritual commitment that two people in love make to each other.

When men and women make the physical commitment without making the emotional and spiritual commitment, one of two detrimental consequences follow. Either the person is burdened with guilt and loss of self-esteem because he knows that he has violated a fundamental part of his nature, or he becomes hardened to the emotional and spiritual aspects of love and separates the physical from its spiritual component. Either result leads to unhappiness.

Marriage

Since the sex act carries with it such responsibility, both physical and emotional, the Bible unequivocally states that it is properly consummated only within the bond of marriage. As already mentioned, sexual intercourse is the ultimate in physical commitment and inter-dependence between a man and a woman. Marriage, in essence, is the commitment of a man and a woman to share the consequences of the sex act as well as the consequences of life in general. Thus in marriage the responsibility of parenthood, establishing a home, making a contribution to society and of fulfilling each other sexually is shared. Because of the responsibility involved, God approves of sexual intercourse only within the spiritual commitment of marriage.

Again the Bible is explicit. Sexual intercourse outside the commitment of marriage is not condoned but sexual relationships within marriage are exalted. When Jesus was asked about divorce, He answered by talking about marriage. In His answer He implied that it was God's plan that a man and woman should leave father and mother and "cleave" to one another. This "cleave" implies not only permanency but intimacy.

The apostle Paul in First Corinthians 7:1-9 deals pointedly with the marriage relationship. He states, "Do not deny yourselves to one another, except when you agree upon a temporary abstinence in order to devote yourselves to prayer; afterwards you may come together again . . ."

Sex is not only permissible in marriage but is a natural part of it. There should be no guilt or shame surrounding the expression of sex between man and wife. Again as the writer of Hebrews says, "Marriage is honorable and the marriage bed undefiled."

Sex As a Servant, Not a Master

Sexual feelings are the product of complex mechanisms surrounded by strong emotions. One reason why the Bible compels the Christian to control his sexual drives is that, if allowed, they will become master instead of the servant God intended them to be. Two young people clawing at each other in the back seat of an automobile, temporarily oblivious to the world around them and unmindful of the consequences of what is about to happen, have become slaves to their sexual urges. A man and woman who rush into marriage without really getting to know each other have become slaves to sex.

When it becomes master, sex is destructive of personality, family, and even the joy that sexual excitement promises. Everyday experience, as well as the Bible, teaches that uncontrolled sexual expression is destructive while sexual expression within the guidelines of the Bible produces fulfillment. Thus almost all societies, pagan and civilized, have seen fit to set up certain rules for the expression of sex. Certainly not all societies limit sex to marriage, but they all realize that sex is such a powerful force that some control is necessary.

Thus the problem of sexual control boils down to whether we will control our sexual impulses or the sexual impulses will control us. As Dr. Henry Bowman, noted marriage authority at the University of Texas quips in his book, *Marriage for Moderns,* "No really intelligent person will burn a cathedral to fry an egg, even to satisfy a ravenous appetite."

To put sex in its proper place as a servant rather than a master requires control of sexual impulses. While some moderns wishfully suggest that sexual restraint prior to marriage endangers health, there is no medical evidence that continence is injurious to health or impairs future sexual capacity; or that previous sexual experience makes one a better husband or wife. (See Chapter 14 for more on this.)

Some misunderstand what psychology teaches about sexual repression. Research has shown that "repressed" sex is dangerous. "Repressed" is a technical term that refers to the process by which a person submerges conflicts, wishes, and dreams into his subconscious (usually at a very early age) so that they can come before the conscious mind only in a disguised form. For example, repression may occur when a toddler is scolded or whipped for handling his genitals. Frequently frightened in this manner, he will bury his sexual thoughts rather than deal with them openly. Such repression is often harmful if not crippling. The previous example of June (the school teacher who suppressed her true sexual feelings and submerged her sexual emotions into her work, but in the end became bitter) illustrates how repression works.

When teenagers or young adults are engaged in resisting a conscious desire, they are in no danger of creating a repression. They are very aware of sexuality and the more they seek to control and master their impulses, the more aware of sex they become. Such a struggle does not harm but preserves peace of mind and future happiness.

Many Christian young people are committed to a high standard of sexual conduct because of their own family experience and their allegiance to Christ. They are not likely to become involved in irresponsible sexual actions, not because they don't have sexual feelings, but because of their understanding of the rewards of controlling them.

But as a physician, I am concerned about the large numbers of young people from Christian homes who do become slaves to their own sexuality. Illegitimate pregnancy, premature marriage, and sexual unhappiness all too often involve children from Christian homes. I believe this occurs as often as it does because in too many homes children and young people receive little help in understanding their sexual feelings and desires. Christian young people need a Christian sex education.

The Bible tells us why God ordained sex. It also tells us that the same God who warns us of the dangers of misusing sex also understands the depths of feelings that surrounds our sexual nature. He understands those who stumble in this area and forgives sexual sins just as He forgives lying, stealing, cheating, or murder. He knows the importance and complexity of sex and in His great providence, deals clearly with sex in the Bible.

The noted philosopher, Dr. T. B. Maston, states in the *Baptist Student*, "It should be remembered, however, that God's commandments are not the arbitrary requirements of some oriental despot. They come from the God who created man and knows what is best for man and for the society of men. We can be sure that His 'you shall not commit adultery' is for our own good. This commandment, as is true of all others, is in harmony with the nature He has given us. No commandment of His, when properly understood will be burdensome."

Questions For Discussion and Thought

1. "My virginity was such a burden to me that I just went out to get rid of it," *Time Magazine* quotes a college student as saying. Discuss why she might feel this way.
2. Does the increased sexual permissiveness today call for more responsibility on the part of young people? How can we as parents help them make responsible decisions about sex?
3. Why is sexual intercourse sanctioned by the Bible only in marriage?
4. "All societies, pagan and civilized, have seen fit to set up certain rules for the expression of sex." Why do you think societies have found such rules necessary?

PART THREE

◆

SEX AMONG THE INNOCENTS

Chapter 5

Sex Starts Here

Rachel Wharton, six months pregnant and showing it, was concerned about what to tell Micky, her five-year-old son, about the pregnancy.

"Mommy, why are you getting fat?" Micky asked, looking up from his tinker toy project.

"We are going to have another baby at our house," his mother replied.

"Does the baby live inside of you?" he asked, now obviously interested.

Hardly waiting for answers to his previous questions, Micky bombarded his mother with one question after another.

"Will it be a boy or a girl?"

"How will it get out?"

"Can I have a baby?"

Many adults are surprised that such questions come from a five-year-old. Often adults think that interest in sex suddenly springs into existence during the teenage years. But as every parent soon discovers, curiosity about sexual matters does not suddenly blossom at adolescence but is present throughout childhood.

Curiosity about sex in young children is a manifestation of their maturing interest in themselves and their environment. As such, it should be accepted in much the same way parents accept the child's curiosity about other things. The interest of each child varies according to his age, the sort of home and cultural environment in which he lives, his relationship to his parents, his intelligence and personality.

A child's sexual attitudes and concepts are determined by how the parents live, think, and answer his questions. Critical concepts about love, the relationship of men and women, and the home are formed as the child observes and interacts with his parents.

By understanding the phases of sexual interests and stages of development through which each child passes, the parent can aid him in finding the right answers to the right questions at the right times.

Love Is Basic

In human terms, sex is an integral part of love. It is an expression of a desire to find meaning and worth in another individual. In our society, however, we are bombarded with the idea that sex can be separated from love. Sex without the commitment of love is exploited in advertising, the movies, and the press. Thus if children are to conceive of sex in its proper relationship to love and marriage, they must learn from their parents.

The love of a husband and wife for each other is the essence of good sex education. In a home where love is abundant, the young child gradually learns to give love in return. First loving his mother and father and other members of his family, he later learns to love others outside the family and finally, he is prepared for the love that leads to marriage.

Love is shown both by discipline and by letting go at the proper time. Some parents mistake permissiveness for love and set few or inconsistent limits for their children. But real love will mean firm limits when the child's actions interfere with his own safety and well-being or the rights of others. It is love that prevents a child from playing with fire or a dangerous tool such as a sharp knife. It is love that disciplines a child when he tramples in the neighbor's flower beds or steals a toy from the child next door. If he is not taught to respect the rights of others, he eventually will be an outcast and disliked by his peers.

We as parents also show love for our children by being able to let them go at the right moment. A mother shows her love by letting her baby feed himself when he is ready instead of "helping" him so much that he loses interest in doing it for himself. It is difficult for some parents to accept the fact that their growing child is finding more meaningful relationships outside the family. The young child, completely dependent on parents for life, is soon the teenager searching for identity and independence. It takes a lot of love to see our son off on his first camping trip when he is nine years old, or to see a daughter off on her first real date at fifteen. But learning such independence is the essence of maturity.

A child who grows up in a family which has little time or inclination to love and play with him is likely to be suspicious, overly demanding and live in fear and dependency. As a teenager, he has a difficult time dating and building the attitudes that lead to a happy life. The evidence indicates that a child born to a loving devoted family goes into marriage with a better chance of happiness than a child whose first steps were taken in an impersonal, unloving world. Love should be given as naturally as food, clothing, and shelter and is more important than all three. It is not something the child should have to demand or earn.

A happy loving home is the first step to a healthy understanding of sex. Without it all efforts of sex education will be incomplete.

Both Mother and Father Are Important

The example we parents set will determine what our children's attitude toward sex will be. It is natural for children to copy their parents whom they love and respect. In homes where the parents' love for each other and their children is expressed in mutual consideration and respect, the children are likely to grow up giving such love. If parents avoid mentioning sex and treat it as something dirty, the children are likely to adopt the same attitude. If parents use coarse and vulgar language in reference to sex, the child will probably speak of sex in the same way.

In setting an example, both mother and father are important. Both parents should be involved with the child in all aspects of child rearing and this is particularly true of sex education. Both boys and girls learn things from each parent that they cannot learn from the other.

From his father a boy learns what it means to be a man — how a man walks, talks and plays. He also learns from his father how to act toward women. A son who sees his father being courteous — opening doors, carrying packages, not hitting back — will likely adopt the same habits. A son whose father treats women disrespectfully is likely to do the same. From his mother a son learns what women are like — how they feel, how they laugh, and how they cry. A boy who has a chance to understand his mother will likely grow into a man who understands women in general. A mother can do much to build up her son's concept of his masculinity through proper guidance and appropriate compliment.

A girl looks to her mother for a feminine model. Her attitude toward her own femininity as well as toward other women will largely mirror her mother's. From her mother the daughter also learns poise, self-confidence and feminine ideals. From her father, a girl forms an opinion of what men are like. The girl who witnesses her father being harsh and inconsiderate to her mother tends to see all men that way. On the other hand, if she can respect her father as a man, she is more likely to respect and understand men when she becomes an adult.

In relaying factual information to young children, both

parents are important. Either parent can effectively teach the preschooler the proper names for different parts of his body. As the child grows older, it becomes more appropriate for the parent of the same sex to relay sexual information. It might be best for the father to explain the elements of sexual intercourse to his preadolescent son, although some mothers might be able to do it. In the same manner, a mother can best tell her growing daughter about menstruation. However, sex education should not be completely segregated. If necessary, mothers should feel comfortable in telling their sons about intercourse. Fathers should also feel able to relay the same information to their daughters, if asked.

Also, there are many things older children can learn about sex from the parent of the opposite sex. A teenage girl can learn best from her father about those things that arouse and attract boys and how to handle the boy once he is attracted. From his mother the teenage boy can best learn how girls feel and expect to be treated.

From the relationship of their mother and father, children form concepts of what marriage is like. If they see constant friction and arguments between their parents and only rare displays of love, they are likely to have a low opinion of what marriage has to offer and in the end seek sexual gratification outside the bond of marriage. On the other hand, if they see their mother and father genuinely giving and loving, then they, themselves, will see marriage as a desirable goal.

Probably the one best lesson in sex education occurs when a father affectionately hugs his wife and gives her a kiss in front of the children. This will do more to give them a wholesome attitude toward sex than any number of words.

Attitudes Toward the Body

Attitudes toward the body and attitudes toward sex are intertwined. Since we must live with both the sex drive and the body, it behooves us to have a concept of both with which we are comfortable. When we fail to do this, mental anguish results.

When Minerva was three, her mother found her sitting on the potty feeling of her vagina.

"Dirty, dirty," her mother shouted angrily and spanked her with a shoe. "Don't ever do that again," she warned.

When Minerva was twelve, her mother wouldn't let her wear a gym suit in the junior high gym class because "it was sinful to show off the body." Minerva could not help but adopt these attitudes of her mother. As a young lady, she longed to be pretty like her friends but she felt guilty about wearing make-up. After marriage, she could not bring herself to even dress or undress in the presence of her husband. She could not have satisfactory sexual relations until she undertook a long period of counseling.

Minerva shows us how one's attitudes toward the body and one's sexual attitudes are interwoven. Confusion about the body will inevitably lead to confusion about sex.

C. S. Lewis in his delightful little book, *The Four Loves,* states that there are three possible attitudes which we can take toward our body:

The first is the pagan concept which states that the body is the prison, or tomb of the soul. Terms such as "sack of dung," "food for worms," "shameful," "a source of nothing but temptation" are used to describe the body. Since sexuality is inevitably tied to the body, sex is considered "shameful." This is, of course, the attitude expressed by Minerva's mother.

The concept that the mind and body, or soul and body, can be separated and that the "flesh" is evil stems from Greek philosophy; it is not Christian or biblical. But regretfully, this pagan concept has at times crept into Christian life and influenced the church's attitude toward the body and sex.

At the other extreme are those who glorify the body

to the point of almost worshiping it. They spend endless time and energy in grooming, body building programs, and nature foods. Physical signs of health and fertility are seen as ultimate goals. One's own body and that of his partner along with the technical skills of intercourse become the object of devotion rather than the spiritual and emotional relationships of two people.

Then there are those who attempt to put the body in its proper perspective. They see the body as neither causing good or evil but realize that it can be used by its owner for either. Saint Francis of Assisi said it best when he called the body "brother ass." As C. S. Lewis says, in *The Four Loves,* "Ass is exquisitely right because no one in his senses can either revere or hate a donkey. It is a useful, sturdy, lazy, obstinate, patient, lovable and infuriating beast; deserving now the stick and now the carrot, both pathetically and absurdly beautiful." That is the body; there is no reason to be ashamed of it, neither is there any reason to worship it.

If in the process of sex education parents can convey to their children this matter-of-fact attitude toward the body, they will be doing their children a great service. Children need to be taught to respect and take care of their bodies and not to misuse them. Their happiness and security will be increased by doing so. They should not be made ashamed of any part of their bodies or any of the body's functions. After all, God made the body as it is. Genesis states that Adam and Eve "were both naked, the man and his wife, and they were not ashamed" (Gen. 2:25). On the other hand, our children should not become so enthralled with their own bodies or so preoccupied with physical gratification that they lose sight of the importance of emotional and spiritual relationships.

Parents Need to Feel Comfortable

Mary was one of a group of fourteen-year-olds who were discussing sex with their club leader.

"I could never talk to my mother about this," Mary sighed. "She'd be so uncomfortable."

Children are extremely sensitive and they sense another's uneasiness or embarrassment. Whether a parent looks on sex as a wholesome, creative aspect of life or sees it as something to be hushed up, or sees it mostly as a topic for tantalizing jokes, children are sure to catch and retain parental attitudes. Thus to help our children acquire the proper concepts of sex, we need to understand our own feelings about it.

Parents are often told that they should be "natural" when talking to their children about sex. While parents do need to be frank and honest, they should not be aloof or unemotional. As a matter of fact, that would not be natural. The most natural thing about sex is the emotional involvement that everyone has in and with it. So when we talk to our children about sex we should not control our emotions to the point that we hide them. Rather, we should let them know and see that we feel strongly about this intimate area of our lives. Parents should not be so "natural" that their children come to think sex concerns only facts or that it can be separated from love.

When children come to us with questions, they want the facts. But they also want to find out what we think about these facts. Children come to us because they trust us; they will continue trusting until we as parents give them reason not to. Whatever the question, words will not be enough unless the child can clearly tell how the parent feels.

Some parents are reluctant to talk about sex with their children because they think such a discussion may suggest to the child the sexual character of the adult. And parents are often strangely uncomfortable when they think their children will find out the truth about them. If the parent describes coitus to the child, then there is the risk that the child will make the correct guess that his parents engage in it.

This hesitancy on the part of the parent to express his sexuality to the child is natural, but it should not get in the way of real dialogue. If parents have come to grips with their own sexuality and are not ashamed of it, then they will not be ashamed to talk to their child about sex. But if they still have some unresolved guilt feelings about their own personality as a sexual being, they will have difficulty in being frank and honest with their children.

A Maze of Rules

Parents need not feel that their success or failure as parents hinges on doing everything right — saying the right thing at the right time or being completely free of sexual hangups. But some parents do feel guilty because they think they are not rearing their child in the best way possible. They read innumerable books and listen to endless authorities. Confused by a maze of rules and regulations, they live in constant fear of inflicting psychic trauma on their child.

These parents need to realize that a certain amount of psychic trauma is the inevitable lot of every child. A youngster growing up without some rebuffs is ill prepared for adult life — for certain traumatic experiences are part of all our environments. Parents should be open to new ideas and methods, but they should not feel pressured to be perfect by the authorities, including this one. One or two unfortunate experiences during childhood — getting their feelings hurt, or being supplied with some misinformation — will not ruin a child for life. Not one decision or action on the parent's part determines what the children shall be. It is the sum total of their actions, words, and attitudes that shapes the personality and attitudes of their offspring.

There are wide variations in how parents can meet

the challenge of sex education. If parents have a whole-some attitude about sex, are comfortable with their own sexual feelings and have a modicum of factual informa-tion, their children's development should be healthy even if the parent occasionally miscues and gives the wrong information, or gives it too soon or too late, or simply fail to communicate at all. The sum total of the parent-child relationship will overshadow the occasional miscue.

Perfect instruction is no more necessary in sex educa-tion than it is in anything else. Parents don't know all there is to know about cars, TV and flowers — yet they teach their children much about them. The same with sex education: they don't have to know everything. The important fact is how they tell what they do know and what attitude they express about the questions be-ing asked by the children.

In summary, the child's attitudes toward sex starts right in the home with what his parents feel, say and do.

Questions For Discussion and Thought

1. What are some of the forces in our society which in-fluence young people to separate love from sex?
2. How can we as parents counter these forces and teach our children that sex and love are integrally inter-woven?
3. Which of your parents were most responsible for telling you about sex? Why?
4. Which of you parents, mother or father, has been most active in conveying sex information to your chil-dren? Why?
5. Which of the concepts of the body did you learn as a child? Do you still have that same basic concept?
6. Do you feel comfortable in discussing sex with your mate? With your children? How can you become more comfortable?

Chapter 6

Facts Aren't Enough

Four-year-old Susan was quite interested when she was told that a new baby was growing inside of her mother's body. After her baby brother, John, was born she watched her mother bathe him; she helped with the diapering by fetching clean diapers and holding the pins. Her mother made no attempt to hide John's anatomy from Susan who occasionally asked questions about why Johnny was different from her. When she asked why John had a penis and she didn't, her mother explained that John had a penis because he was a boy. She explained that instead of a penis, Susan had a vagina like other girls. Sex information and attitudes came gradually to Susan through day-to-day experiences as her questions were answered honestly.

This is the way sex education should be. The home is the best place for it, the parents are the most ideal teachers and the best method is that of daily living.

The home is the best place to convey sex information to children because it can be done individually and integrated naturally into all of life's experiences. Parents know their children better than anyone else — they know their maturity level as well as what language they understand. Also, parents are more likely to inject the moral aspects of sexuality that are so important to the development of a wholesome view of sex. This does not mean that information about sex should not be taught at church and at school; they certainly should. But sex education at church and school should be complementary to what the child receives at home, not given in place of it.

Although parents are the ideal ones to teach their children about sex, many parents feel uncomfortable and inadequate to do the job. Some feel too emotional or too embarrassed to talk to their children about sex while others feel that they "don't know enough." However, to be successful, parents do need to feel comfortable and must know at least a smattering of the basic facts.

Actually, many parents are surprised by the degree of comfort with which they can talk with their children about sex once they open the door of communication. In doing so, they feel even more adequate as parents.

For the communication between parent and child to be effective, it must begin during the early years and continue as the child grows. Parents can be sure that if they have been silent or inhibited about sex they cannot expect their twelve-year-old suddenly to start opening his mind to them. It is also harder for the parent to start talking openly to his children when he has been strangely silent in the past.

Many authorities agree that sex education is only as good as the attitudes it develops in the child about family life, marriage, the body, and how love is expressed. This kind of learning extends throughout childhood. Obviously these attitudes are learned primarily in the home. If facts were all that there was to sex education, then the school or church could do the job alone, but they are not.

Facts alone are not enough.

What to Teach

This brings us to the important question: "What should be taught in the process of sex education?"

There are two approaches one can take in teaching

about sex: Emphasis on the anatomy and physiology of sex (the plumbing approach), or emphasis on attitudes and morals. The plumbing approach focuses on the egg, the sperm, how they get together, and what happens after they collide. In the attitudinal approach, attitudes, interpersonal relationships, and morality are emphasized. Certainly both aspects should be integrated in a proper sex education. A child's growing curiosity demands that he know the facts and if he doesn't learn them at home he will learn them elsewhere under less desirable circumstances. At the same time the child needs and wants to know how to put the facts in the proper perspective of human relationships.

With most topics, a child's questions are given a matter-of-fact reply. But when his curiosity touches on his origin or his body parts, parents often become embarrassed, annoyed, or shocked and create an atmosphere that precludes further discussion. But to a child of any age, sex as a subject is not separated from the rest of life. The older toddler is curious about his body and this includes his genitals. He is no more or less concerned about his penis than he is about his nose. He only becomes more concerned about it when adults act differently when the penis is touched or mentioned than when the nose is the object of one's curiosity.

In the same way, the preschool child is interested in "Where did I come from?" By this he means that he is interested in who made him as well as how did he get out of his mother's abdomen. He does not become more interested in the later unless adults become embarrassed and refuse to answer his questions about how he got out. The adolescent boy or girl is not only interested in how sexual intercourse happens but they are interested in what it means to be a boy or girl, not just from the biological point of view, but also from the spiritual and social aspects as well.

What to Teach

To prepare adequately to teach their children about sex, parents need to learn some of the basic facts about the human body. Unfortunately, many parents are not well educated in this because they had poor or no instruction when they were growing up. Husbands and wives should talk to each other about the facts. They can attend PTA meetings and other groups where the subject is discussed. They should talk to their family physician. If he does not have the time to discuss the facts, he will often be able to give them some free material on the subject, recommend some good books, and refer them to a specialist in sex education if necessary. Fortunately, there are many good books and manuals available to the parent describing the anatomical and physiological facts.

You are fortunate if you are among those few parents who have a good grasp of the facts, thanks to your own parents, school or college training.

The use of the correct terms for genitals and body functions will make it easier for the parent to converse with the child about sex. Parents can easily master the use of the correct terms such as penis, buttocks, rectum, vagina, etc. If you were reared without the benefit of these correct terms they may be unfamiliar and you may have to begin gradually to use them.

Mothers, for instance, continually converse with their children. At bath time, such events as this occur: "Now let's wash those dirty hands. Turn around and I will wash your back." The alert parent can continue in a natural way, "Now let's wash your penis. We need to pull the foreskin back like this so that we can get it real clean."

Many mothers dread the day when they must sit down and explain menstruation to their preteen daughter. However, if both mother and daughter are conversant with the proper terms, the job will be much easier and less frightening for both mother and daughter. In fact, it can be a stimulating and mutually rewarding experience if they both come to it with the proper vocabulary and attitudes.

A glossary of the more common and important terms is found at the end of the book. Now would be a good time to stop and review the terms and their proper definitions.

Preparing oneself to teach the attitudinal and moral aspect of sex is a different matter. Attitudes and morals will primarily be determined by the parents' background and religious training. Parents should creatively evaluate what they feel and think about sex for two reasons. First, the parent needs to know what he really feels about sex and why. Secondly, parents should evaluate what they believe. They need to see if some of their ingrained attitudes and concepts are really true. Particularly, the Christian must determine if his concept of sexuality is compatible with what the Bible really teaches about sex or has it been distorted by Greek, Puritan, or Victorian ideas that are basically non-Christian?

When Should Sex Be Taught

A mother brought her thirteen-year-old boy to see the pediatrician. "Doctor," she began, "Richard's growing up now, and we haven't taught him anything about sex. Would you tell him the facts of life?"

As we learned in Chapter 1, Richard will by this time have absorbed a good dose of facts — mostly distorted facts — from his friends and the bathroom walls. It will take much more than a once-for-all doctor-patient talk, or father-son chat, to get him straightened out. Sexual feelings and attitudes do not suddenly occur for the first time when a child's sex organs are ready for reproduction. Sex interest begins in infancy and grows as the child grows. His interests and needs are different at different ages. To be effective, sex education should begin in infancy and be integrated into all of the child's life experiences in language he understands.

A parent may legitimately ask, "Can't you teach too much too soon?" Throughout this book, emphasis is put on answering the child's questions whenever he asks them. However, this certainly does not mean that parents should unload the whole story at one sitting. It does not mean that a parent should give all the details of birth to a five-year-old or give an explicit description of sexual intercourse to a seven-year-old.

There is a proper time in the child's development to introduce different topics and facts. Although the appropriate time will vary from child to child depending on his mental abilities, emotional stability, and curiosity, we can have a general idea of what is proper for a given age.

Information given too soon may be meaningless to the child, or, worse, provoke anxiety. On the other hand, information given too late leads the child to believe that his parents do not care about his feelings or that they are ignorant; or worse still, it leads the child to seek information under undesirable and shaky circumstances. It may well lead the child to unhealthy experimentation. For instance, the five-year-old who does not have a clear understanding of why the sexes are different may peek into bathrooms or explore another child's anatomy to see what the difference is. Such lack of information often leads teenagers into heavy petting or premature sexual intimacy.

When do you tell your child about sex? What do you tell when? The best guide is your child's own questions. When the child asks about a sexual matter answer him in language appropriate to his age. Section three of this book deals in detail with what is appropriate language for each stage of development.

How to Teach About Sex

Sex education should be a natural part of the child's day-to-day life, not set aside as a special course of study. This means that the child learns about sex as he learns about other things, when his curiosity leads him to ask questions. When a four-year-old asks what candy is made of, he is likely to get a matter-of-fact reply in words he can understand. When he asks where babies come from he deserves the same type of honest answer. Because of the child's natural curiosity, questions will come if the lines of communication are kept open.

The first step in being a good teacher is to be a good listener. It is important to know what the child is asking. What he is asking may be more — or less — than the parent thinks. One five-year-old asked his father where he came from. The father, thinking that this was a good time to give him the facts of life, began a long, serious discussion. At the finish of the dissertation, the son replied, "Okay, Dad, but where did I come from. Rick came from Utah. Did I come from there too?"

To find out what your child is concerned about when asking a question, you may reply in a puzzled manner, "What do you mean?" This will allow him to provide you with a basis for his question and will help you see just what his understanding of the subject is. It will often help you to see if he has any misconceptions that you will need to clear up before you actually get down to the business of answering the question.

Some parents say, "But my child never asks any questions about sex." While unusual, some children for reasons of their own seem to smother their own curiosity. Faced with such a situation, the parents should look at their own attitudes to see if they discourage questions. If this is so, it is best to admit it and seek ways to open the door of communication with the child. A marriage, a pregnancy or a birth are natural events which can be used as a door opener.

What about using examples in nature (such as the family dog having pups) as a method of teaching about sex? With the prechooler, such examples are likely to be more confusing than helpful. Children at this age have a difficult time separating fact from fantasy. With the elementary school age child, examples from the plant and animal kingdom may help him understand the scientific basis of reproduction. But care should be taken to make sure the child understands that there are qualitative differences in human and animal sexuality; that there is more to human sexuality than just mating.

What about giving a child books on sex to read? Some parents feel that just handing a book to their child is a sufficient sex education in itself. Hopefully we have already shown that there is much more to sex education than facts gleaned from books and the attitudes parents convey directly to their children are quite important. Certainly parents cannot know all there is to know about sex and will need to refer to books and other references for help. With the grade school child, the parent and child can look at books and pictures together with the parent explaining their meaning. It is appropriate to give the adolescent books to read on his own for he is capable and interested in independent investigation. But even at this age, the book should not be a substitute for an available and concerned parent.

Questions For Discussion and Thought

1. Where did you receive the majority of your sex education? At home? At school? At church? On the street? From your parents? From teachers? From your friends?

2. Where are your children receiving the majority of their sex information?

3. What resources are available in your community to

help you as a parent better educate your children about sex?

4. At what age did you learn the facts of birth? The facts of copulation?

5. Do your children know about these facts? At what age did they learn? From whom?

6. Do your children ask questions about sexual matters: frequently, occasionally, never? If never, why do you think this is so?

Chapter 7

◆

"I've Been Wondering . . ."

This chapter discusses several miscellaneous, but important questions that parents often ask concerning sex and their children. The concepts dealt with here are crucial at all stages of growth and development, thus they are presented together as an introduction to the next section of the book which discusses each stage of development separately.

Developing a Sense of Privacy

Privacy, valued as a right, is more and more difficult to find in our day of over-population and thin walled apartments. Parents do their children a valuable service if they teach them early to enjoy their own privacy, and respect that of others. This usually is not difficult. At about six years of age many children develop a need for privacy and modesty. This is healthy and should be encouraged. Preschoolers can be taught to respect family members' privacy while dressing or in the bathroom. They can also be taught to respect closed bathroom and bedroom doors and to knock before entering.

However, a child learns best by example and parents should give him the same courtesy when he requests it. A child of four or five who is able to dress and care for himself at the toilet is best allowed to do so alone unless help is requested. In the same manner, the best way to teach him to respect mother's and daddy's closed bedroom door is to respect his and to knock before entering. In fact, this could and should be a family rule.

It is probably best for brothers and sisters not to bathe or sleep together after the age of five. While casual observation of each other made during the early years is not harmful and may even be desirable, the prolonged contact of sleeping or bathing together will likely produce problems. One mother who had let her daughter and son bathe together found that she had trouble breaking the habit when the children were five years old. This habit, if carried on long enough, might not only inhibit the child from developing a sense of privacy, but could cause premature sexual stimulation.

It is so important to the happiness of the whole family for the parents to have a wholesome and uninhibited sex life that every effort should be made to insure privacy and peace in the parental bedroom. It is undesirable for children to share bedrooms with their parents. They see and hear more than adults think and certainly most parents could not relax in the sexual roles with a child in the room, even though sound asleep.

Parents should not allow children to sleep with them except in special temporary situations, such as illness. This habit is not only harmful for the child but for the marriage relationship as well. As for the child, this habit inhibits the child's development of independence. It is also dangerous in that the child literally comes between the parents, physically and sometimes emotionally. It is best for the happiness of the family and the growth of the child that he learn to sleep alone and respect the privacy of all family members.

Nudity

Closely allied with the question of privacy is that of nudity. Some parents, determined to disavow a Victorian heritage, use their own nudity as a vehicle to demonstrate the difference between the sexes. This is a practice that is probably more confusing than illuminating to the child. To see a much larger, hairy genital clarifies little and with looking, there often comes the wish to touch, a request understandably embarrassing to most parents.

Fathers and sons can dress together and need not hide their nudity; so can mothers and daughters. But it is not advisable for mothers and sons, or fathers and daughters to dress in the presence of one another. While a child's occasional intrusion, accidental or on purpose, may be tolerated, such intrusions should not be encouraged nor should the home be run like a nudist colony. Seeing grown-ups of the opposite sex nude may produce anxieties with which the child cannot cope.

Children are curious about the human body. Sometimes a child, particularly the four- or five-year-old, may try to enter the bathroom with his parent. The parent can respond by saying, "I know you want to know what the adult body looks like. But when I go to the bathroom, I want to be alone. I will be glad to answer any questions you may have."

Gender Differences

Parents should encourage the boy or girl to act appropriate to his or her sex and discourage actions that are not. While it is normal for some girls to be "tomboys," such actions should not be encouraged. Boys, particularly young boys, may occasionally dress as a girl putting on a skirt or a dress. Such a boy should not be laughed at or ridiculed, but gently informed that boys do not dress like that and he should be encouraged in more masculine actions.

During the grade school years children need opportunity to develop a close relationship with the parent of the same sex. It is healthy for mother and daughter to do girl things together (sewing, shopping, cooking) and for father and son to engage in masculine activities (baseball, hunting, repair jobs).

This is particularly important for the boy. In our society boys are engulfed by females. They spend the preschool years at home with their mothers or in a nursery school with female attendants. When they start to school their teachers, often including principals and PE teachers, are female. In the past the boy worked side by side with his father in the field or shop. Thus he had a natural opportunity to identify with the masculine role. But today it is not appropriate or practical for sons to accompany their fathers to offices and factories. Today such closeness requires a special effort by the father. The best gift a father can give his son is some of his time.

Sex Play

It is not uncommon for children aged four to nine years to participate in play that is plainly sexual in nature. This may occur in the guise of innocent appearing games such as "doctor" or "nurse" which involves the removing of clothing and intimate touching of each other. Little girls may hide in the bathroom and giggle about toilet functions, little boys may repeat enticing jokes which they have overheard. Sometimes both boys and girls invent peeping games in which they show off interesting parts of their anatomy. "I'll show you mine if you will show me yours," is a common invitation.

One reason why children engage in sex play is to satisfy their curiosity about what the other sex looks like and to see what their own emerging sex feelings mean. But sex play does not answer these questions — it only confuses the child; and such sex play is harmful to children because it burdens them with guilt while it does not satisfy their needs.

A second reason why children engage in sex play is that they are overstimulated sexually and seek to act on feelings unnaturally aroused. A lack of basic sex information plus the excessive sexual stimulation found in advertising, TV and magazines place the American youngster in a vulnerable position. Sex play, rather than cooling the emotions produced by this stimulation, only frustrate it.

Even the most enlightened parents are often at a loss in dealing with this situation. They are torn between shaming and spanking or trying to act as if they did not see the sex play. However, an adult can best handle such situations at home, school or camp by calmly, but firmly, making it plain that such behavior is not tolerated. He can say, "I know that you were undressing each other. That is not allowed in this house. If there is anything you want to know about how people look, come ask me and we will talk about it. But no touching or undressing."

The parent can follow up on this later when emotions have cooled. For example, the father can say to his son, "I know that you are curious about what a girl's body looks like. Let's look at some diagrams and you can ask me your questions."

On these matters the parent should not compromise — the child should understand that secret sex play is not allowed. But he should also know that no question asked of the parent is taboo. The best way to prevent excessive sex play among children is to keep communication open between parent and child. If the child knows that he can get answers from his parents he is less likely to experiment. By being calm but firm it is possible to limit the child's experimentation without harming his interest in wholesome sex and love.

Bad Language

Often parents ask, "What do we do when Johnny brings home dirty words?"

Parents should learn to expect this. Often innocently,

occasionally to create a sensation, children will try out swear words and crude sexual terms at home. A four- or five-year-old may bring home objectionable words because he heard some older youngsters use them. With the grade schooler, using such language is taken as a badge of being "grown up." Nothing is really gained by the parent acting shocked or horrified — this simply makes the use of the words more exciting to the child. But this does not mean that the parent should ignore what the child is doing or saying. Let him understand that the words are no surprise and that you know what he means. While harsh punishment is not indicated, the parent can, in no uncertain terms, let the child know that such language is not allowed and its use is bad manners like nose picking.

Incidentally, if it is apparent that the child does not know the meaning of his new word, the parent should explain it to him plainly, even though this may be painful for the parent. Often when the child knows the real meaning of what he is saying, the word drops from his vocabulary.

Pornography

Pornography is difficult to define. Even the Supreme Court and Congress cannot arrive at an acceptable definition. But for our purposes, pornography can be defined as any obscene, immodest written or pictorial material which is deliberately designed to feed perverted sexual desires. With the inability of the courts to define pornography, the presence of such material in magazine racks, book stores and specialty shops has become commonplace in our society. There is no doubt that obscene and lewd material is easily accessible to children as well as adults. Thus, the chance of our children coming in contact with some form of pornography, accidentally or deliberately, is fairly great.

It is not known to what extent, if any, pornography is dangerous. Some claim that it leads to excessive sexual appetite, while others claim that the use of such material serves as a harmless sexual outlet. There is no real proof for either of these views. However, we as Christian parents should be concerned about pornography for another reason. Regardless of its other effects, such material will convey to children and young adolescents distorted and perverted concepts of what sex is all about. Often so-called "art" pictures sex as the ultimate goal in life and holds women up as nothing more than sexual machines to be used for the gratification of men. Pornography often pictures all women as being nymphomaniacs who are ready to fall in bed, or in the bushes, with the first man who glances at her. Such fallacies and distortions confuse and misguide children. In this sense, it is certainly harmful.

This is not the place to debate the legality and constitutionality of pornography. It is apparent that lewd and obscene materials will continue to be available in our society in one form or another. While parents together and individually should work to prevent or lessen the chances of such material being available to their children, their chances of being successful are not great.

Thus parents need to seek ways to lessen the impact of pornography on their children. The best way to do this is to give your child a clear understanding of male and female anatomy and instill in him from early life the true meaning of sex. A child who has a basic knowledge about sex is less likely to be shocked or influenced by pornography. Also in a family where there has been open communication about sex between the parents and children, the children will likely not try to hide such material if they accidentally discover it. On the other hand, a child who has been kept in the dark about sex is likely to find anything sensuous, including the lewd and obscene, particularly interesting and will devour all such material he or she can find. It is tragic if such material serves as the child's only sex education.

Parents are confused about what to do if they inadvertently discover their child with such material or find it hidden in the child's room. Some parents will be so embarrassed they will ignore it. Others will react in extreme anger. Neither of these approaches is likely to be effective. The best way to handle this situation would be to approach the child quietly without embarrassment and explain that such material is not a reliable source of sex information. You may say, "If you have some question about sex, please ask me. If I don't know the answer, we will find out." You might then offer him an appropriate book about sex to read.

Punishment, embarrassment, shouting and condemnation will do little good and will only drive the child farther underground in search for answers about sex.

Masturbation

Masturbation, or self-stimulation of the genital organs, is a universal habit that sooner or later concerns most parents and children. Parents wonder if their child is weird, sick or doomed for engaging in masturbation. Children often feel both curiosity and guilt about it.

Since masturbation is common to all ages and since there are so many questions about it, the subject will crop up in numerous sections of this book. At this time a general introduction to the nature and consequences of masturbation will be introduced. Questions relating to specific ages will be presented in later chapters.

Kinsey and others who have studied the sex habits of a cross section of our society point out that the majority of people of both sexes engage in some form of masturbation during childhood. However, the very mention of the word "masturbation" often brings on raised eyebrows and gasps of shock. Contrary to popular belief, masturbation does not cause insanity, stunted growth, perversions, feeble-mindedness, or sterility. Nor does it cause acne, dark circles under the eyes, or weakness. In fact there are no known physically damaging effects of masturbation. The fact that almost everyone has masturbated to some degree at some time in his life shows that it is not the destructive habit that it is sometimes made out to be.

Self-manipulation occurs in early childhood, adolescence and adulthood and may have different meanings at different ages. Such manipulation of the genital organs during early childhood, though common, may have little significance. It is natural for infants and toddlers to explore their bodies including their genitals. Although led to such exploration by curiosity they quickly discover that they may get pleasurable sensations by feeling certain parts of the body. Such occasional masturbation is accidental and sporadic. Rarely, frustrated, bored, or nervous children may develop a persistent habit of masturbation as a way to release emotional tension. But in this case, the underlying frustration and anxiety is the real problem, not the masturbation itself. The toddler caught massaging his or her genitals should be gently guided into some interesting activity. Making an issue of the child's actions by spanking, scolding or lecturing, only creates a conscious interest in an act that the child was most likely doing casually. By so doing, parents often make masturbation more attractive to the child.

Masturbation reaches its peak during adolescence at which time it becomes a definitely conscious act whose purpose is the release of sexual tension. The years from puberty to marriage are difficult ones for the adolescent. In both boys and girls, the sexual drive is reaching its peak during adolescence. Since in our society marriage usually does not occur until the late teens or early twenties, the adolescent either must repress his sexual drives, engage in premarital intercourse, or masturbate. Premarital sex, while becoming more and more acceptable in our society is not acceptable to the Christian parent or youth. While some sexual energy can be repressed or sublimated into creative activities, for most teenagers complete repression and sublimation is neither possible nor desirable. Thus occasional masturbation is a frequently used sexual outlet and as such is neither physically or psychologically harmful.

Frequent and compulsive masturbation is a different matter. Such excessive preoccupation with self-gratification often is a way of compensating for failure, anxiety, or feelings of inferiority and inadequacy. Walter, although fifteen years old, was skinny and shy. He longed to date, but he even lacked the courage to ask a girl to the high school football games. He compensated for his lack of gratifying friendships by masturbation. Joan, a junior in high school, not only did not have many dates, she was not doing well in school. She discovered that she could escape all her frustrations by masturbation. In time it became a compulsive habit that she could not easily stop. The usual teenager who has many outlets for his energy and frustrations is not likely to take up compulsive masturbation as a way of life.

Parents should accept occasional masturbation as a phase in the development of normal sexuality and the more desirable method of sexual outlet for the adolescent. But parents are right in not sanctioning persistent, frequent or compulsive self-gratification. Over-indulgence in this area is not emotionally healthy. Self-gratification makes the adolescent less accessible to the influences of parents and peers. Such a person may easily dwell in a world of fantasy created to cover up, but not fulfill his needs. By this, he doesn't have to depend on, or please, anyone but himself.

There are several things a parent can do to prevent the development of compulsive masturbation or to help the child caught up in this habit. He can exert mild pressure against such self-indulgence, not because it is a sickness, but because it is not progressive. The best way to do this is to sit down with the youngster and quietly discuss the situation and explain that masturbation does not doom one to ill health or hell, but that it is a poor substitute for active involvement in friendships and creative activities.

A vigorous life full of physical and social activities will help the adolescent to expand his interests beyond himself. Healthy relationships with the opposite sex through dating will help. Finally, an open door of communication between parent and child in which sexual questions can be discussed frankly will also help clear the air and keep masturbation in proper perspective.

Questions For Discussion and Thought

1. "The best way to teach a child to respect mother and daddy's closed bedroom is to respect the child's own privacy." Do you agree with this statement? Explain your feelings.

2. Young boys of today often lack adult male companionship and a masculine role to identify with. How can we as parents and community help provide this?

3. Our reaction as adults to sex play, bad language and pornography often vacillate between shaming and spanking to quietly ignoring the behavior. Which way do you tend to react? Why? Is there a better way?

4. One author has stated that masturbation is God's gift to the teenager who wants to remain chaste. Do you agree? Why?

PART FOUR

◆

DEVELOPING SEXUALITY

Chapter 8

◆

Infancy and Early Childhood:
Age One to Five

Research in the fields of psychology, medicine, and sociology has shown that the first years of life are the most important ones in the education of the child. One who for any reason is deprived of learning opportunities during these years is severely and sometimes hopelessly behind. In terms of biological time, the degree of change over a chronological time span, development during the first two and a half years of life is more extensive than at any other time. In addition, experiences early in life tend to have more lasting effects upon subsequent development than do experiences in later childhood. For instance, children who spend their early months in an impersonal atmosphere such as orphanages, nursing homes, or hospitals often are unable to form really loving relationships with people later on. This is because a baby's experience with his mother during the critical early months sets the stage for trusting relationships with other people.

A study of neglected youngsters showed that children who do not have the stimulation of love, play, and speech during the early months of their lives tend to do poorly in school compared to others, even though they may receive special help later on. No doubt, a child learns much about himself and his world during the first few years of his life.

Thus, if sex education is to be effective, it must begin early. Actually sex education begins with a child at birth. The way in which a child is held by his mother and father tells him about love; the associations he feels from their muscles, the touch of their fingers, their characteristic body odors, and the characteristic male and female sounds of their voices tells him a great deal about people and their differences. He begins to discriminate emotions by the tone of voice. He begins to learn what love is, not from a dictionary, but from the trust and security he feels in the arms of his parents.

As parents we cannot really choose whether we will give such sex education to our infant. We give it each day in the way we do or do not feel, cuddle and love him.

Learning About Love

Several factors combine very early to direct the infant toward his mother and toward the outside world. The child's relationship with his mother during these early months centers around having his bodily needs met. This is seen most dramatically in feeding. Feeding is important to the child for two reasons. Not only does it provide him with nutrition, but the very act of sucking with its physical closeness to the mother gives a feeling of security and pleasure to the baby. The infant ordinarily will develop a sense of trust and confidence if his parents are reasonably devoted and consistent in caring for him. This relationship must develop if the child is to have any feelings of caring for others in the future. Youngsters who do not experience love and affection in early life often are not able to form deep, loving relationships during adulthood.

Brenda was not wanted by her mother. She received barely enough food to live and received none of the cuddling and warmth usually found in the mother-child relationship. At three years of age, she would not smile or look at anyone in the eyes. She would allow others to pick her up but her body would be rigid and unyielding. Deprived of love as an infant, she did not know how to relate to people later in life.

Dr. Rene Spitz studied hundreds of children in nursing homes and orphanages. He found that those who had received adequate physical care such as feeding and diapering, but did not have the cuddling and affection of motherly love, were withdrawn, sad and unresponsive. Thus, the love that a child receives in infancy determines how that child will be able to give love when he is older.

Learning About the Body

During the first year of life, most babies triple their birth weight and add considerably to their length. After the first year, the growth gradually slows down only to spurt up again at puberty. The baby's rapid growth does not affect all his body parts equally. For example, the newborn baby has a head that is proportionally larger than that of the adult, and his legs are shorter. The various parts of the body go through periods of relatively rapid growth at different times until adult size and proportions are reached.

In both sexes, the reproductive organs are completely formed at birth. But neither the ovaries of the baby girl nor the testes of the baby boy are yet capable of discharging sex cells. The sex organs increase a little in size during the first three years of life, but even then they are only a small fraction of the adult size. However, a young boy can have an erection of the penis. This is likely to happen when he has a full bladder or is stimulated by touch or a tight diaper. It does not mean he is abnormal.

At first, the child's exploration of his body is accidental. He soon discovers his thumb and the pleasure that comes from sucking it. A newborn baby will often suck his thumb when he is only minutes old. This is a pleasure-giving device that infants will continue to use to a greater or lesser degree for years.

Around six months of age, deliberate exploration of the body begins. The baby transfers a toy from one hand to the other, he pulls his ears, tickles his toes, and the boy massages his penis and the girl her vagina. This manipulation is obviously pleasurable to the child. Parents, if not disturbed by the actual manipulation, are frequently shocked by the pleasure the child gets. However, this behavior is an expression of the child's natural inquisitiveness and will not harm him.

Learning Names of Body Parts

Events of the toddler stage more sharply define elements of sexuality. Speech development begins and this helps the toddler in sorting out ideas and feelings. The first words he learns usually include designations for members of the family and body parts; the pronouns "he" and "she" appear at about two years. Attitudes previously taught through looks, gestures, and tones of voice become reinforced by words.

It is fascinating to watch a mother assist her toddler with a bath. As they splash around getting as much water on the floor as on the skin, questions and answers fly back and forth. Nose, ears, and toes are identified and the mother smiles with pride. The young boy spots his penis and grabs it and asks, "What's this?" All too often the mother replies with "ding dong" or some other vulgarized name for penis. The same is true with other parts of the genital organs.

No wonder children pick up street language about sex so easily. The toddler who has been taught that his penis is a "ding dong" will eventually learn from other boys more "grown up" and vulgar names for this most important part of his anatomy. If the child is taught the correct names for his body parts and not to be ashamed of them, he will have no need to pick up the less desirable names. Thus, when a child inquires about a body part, it is best to give the correct name for penis, scrotum, rectum and vagina.

The same is true for body functions also. When a child is given infantile and inappropriate names for body functions, he will soon pick up substitutes. It is best for the parent to call the body functions by their correct names: urinate, bowel movement, etc.

The attitudes a child develops about his body during these early years stick with him forever. Unfortunately a person who has learned to be ashamed of his body as a small child will probably remain disturbed as an adult regardless of how many books he reads or how many facts he learns. Often impotence in men and frigidity in women can be traced to guilt about the body derived from early childhood experiences.

Although we should try to help the child understand his body and give proper names for body parts, we cannot expect him to conceive everything on an adult level.

Three-year-old Jimmy walked up to his father holding his scrotum. "What's this?" he asked.

"That's your scrotum," his father replied. "It contains seed bags. When you grow up and get married, they will help you make babies."

Later Jimmy came running back excited. "Daddy, I can make lots of babies," he explained. "I have two seed bags."

Incidentally, his father gives us a good lesson in sex education. When his son approached him holding his scrotum, he did not shame him, but listened to Jimmy's question. He answered the question frankly and simply, in terms Jimmy could understand. Being a Christian father, he planted the idea that making babies was something reserved for marriage. Thus, as Jimmy grows older and learns that babies are a natural consequence of sexual intercourse, he will know that sexual intercourse is not something to be taken lightly but is reserved for the commitment of marriage. I am not suggesting that this one experience will automatically set such attitudes in Jimmy's young mind. But I do suggest that over the years numerous such experiences will determine Jimmy's wholesome attitude toward his body and sex. This father can have confidence that Jimmy will not hesitate to bring other such questions to him in the future.

Gender Identity

We never think of a baby as just a baby — we think of it as a boy or a girl. It is not an "it" — it is a "he" or "she." The Bible states in Genesis that "God created man in his own image; in the image of God created he him; male and female created he them." Ever since, men and women have been acutely aware of their masculinity and femininity. Each sex and gender has characteristics that separate it from the other. The most obvious fact is the striking difference in sexual organs and sexual functions. Also secondary sex characteristics such as the breasts, hair, and pitch of voice identify one sex from the other in a physical way. But there are also psychological differences. A woman is expected to be tender, a man strong and brave. A woman can show her emotions by crying; a man must hide behind a mask of aloofness.

Although hereditary factors and hormones play a role, the most deciding factor in gender identity is experience. Gender identity is defined "as all those things that a person says or does to disclose himself or herself as being a boy or man, a girl or woman." A gender role is not established at birth but is built up cumulatively through experiences in living, through casual and formal learning, and through explicit guidance and instruction. Thus from a psychological standpoint, a child *learns* to be a boy or a girl.

Susan was born with sex organs that were ambiguous — they resembled neither those of a boy or a girl. The doctor really did not know what sex she was but since the penis was small, she was arbitrarily called a girl. Her birth certificate stated that she was a girl. However, when Susan was three years old, studies were done which showed that her genetic sex was not that of a girl at all, but that she had both an X and Y chromosome. Thus, genetically she was a male.

Should her parents continue to raise Susan as a girl or should they change her name and put her in pants, take away her dolls, and give "him" toy trucks? Psychological tests showed that in every way Susan thought of herself as a girl and her parents wisely decided not to change. Because her parents had treated her as a girl, and in many ways taught her to be a girl, Susan had thoroughly learned to be a girl.

Many studies have shown that gender identity is established by two years of age. After this time, attempts to change the orientation of children who have been placed in the incorrect sex category because of external genital ambiguity have severe psychological consequences. In fact, the child's concept of himself rarely changes even when his hair and clothes are different. The genetic sex is of minor importance in determining what sex a child thinks himself to be; his experience is much more important. Thus a child learns to be a boy or a girl and once this role is learned, it is seldom changed within the child.

How does a child learn this role?

He learns it in many ways. From the start, a boy is usually dressed differently from a girl. Later on, children are told that "You're daddy's boy," or "You're mommy's little girl." Little boys are told that they are rough; little girls are told over and over again that they are cute. Thus, little by little, a child begins to identify himself with one or the other of the parents and begins to mimic the parent's ways and thoughts.

The recognition of sexual differences, like that of differences in skin color and other physical variations, commonly appears between ages two and three. Bathing with siblings and observing the diapering and toileting of other children precipitates a boy's inquiry as to how girls urinate, or a girl's struggle to understand why she has no penis.

Children do not take gender difference for granted. To them it is a great mystery, and they frequently devise great fantasies for explanations. The three- or four-year-old girl may wonder out loud why she does not have a penis. "Did I lose mine?" three-year-old Anne asked when she observed her little brother's penis as her mother changed his diapers. Little boys may ask, "How does Anne pee pee? She doesn't have a place." A little girl may imagine that she lost her penis because of bad behavior or she may believe that she will grow one when she is older. A boy may decide that if a girl can lose hers, he may lose his also.

We should not take such fantasies lightly. These are serious matters to the child. It is helpful to bring such fantasies out in the open. We may say, "Sometimes girls get scared when they see they don't have a penis. Do you ever wonder about this?"

To our son, we may say, "Boys sometimes get worried when they see that little girls don't have a penis. You shouldn't worry about this; girls are different from boys. They are born that way. That is why boys grow up to be fathers and girls grow up to be mothers."

When a child discovers that there are differences in the bodies of boys and girls, it is a good idea to emphasize, rather than minimize, the differences.

To our daughter, we may say, "Because you are a girl, you have a vagina. Girls grow up to be mothers. I'm pleased that you have noticed that girls are made one way and boys another."

To our son, we may reply, "You are a boy and will grow up to be a father. Because you are a boy, you have a penis."

Three-year-old George is beginning to get the right idea. He looks at his penis. "I have a little one. Daddy has a big one. I'm like daddy. Mother and sister are different."

The message as to the sex role the child is to have should be loud and clear because if a child is confused about what sex he is, he will be confused in many other ways.

Toilet Training

All the things a child has learned about love, himself as the sexual being, and his body are tested and re-tested in the process of toilet training. From the standpoint of sexual attitudes, this is one of the most important events of the child's entire development. In this process, a child's attitudes toward his body are, to an extent, fixed. Our child's control of bowels and bladder is another natural step in his development. Acquiring toilet habits means learning to delay defecation and urination temporarily until it can be done in an appropriate place. It differs somewhat from other developmental steps such as sitting up and walking in that it requires more of our assistance and a great deal more patience.

The organs of sex and elimination are so close together that a young child easily gets them confused, and attitudes toward toilet training are easily transferred to the sexual area. Marvin demonstrates how easily three-year-olds can confuse anal and genital structures. For several days he did not have a bowel movement and resisted going to the potty. However, one day his mother insisted that he sit on the pot anyway. While sitting there, he pointed to his testicles and said, "They are mine. I need them." His mother realized that he was afraid that he would pass his testicles in his bowel movement. She reassured him that this certainly would not happen, and he relaxed and his bowel habits reverted to normal.

The main mistake made in toilet training is that of being either too hasty or to harsh. No two children are ready to begin at the same age. No one expects a child to walk before his legs are strong enough to support his body. Similarly, before he can attempt bowel or bladder control, certain muscles and parts of his nervous system must mature to the point that he can exercise some control consciously over them. Thus, toilet training started too early is self-defeating. A child is ready for bowel control around eighteen to thirty months and for urinary control around twenty-four to thirty-six months of age. Accidents, of course, will continue to happen in most children until age five. A child is probably ready to begin developing toilet habits when he is able to walk by himself, has arrived at some regularity in his bowel movements, and has some way of letting his parent know he is uncomfortable.

A child's need for approval makes him try to live up to his mother's wishes for him. If she expects adult-like toilet habits from him when he is not yet capable of them, he will become disappointed in his inability to please her. He may try very hard at first, then sensing his mother's disappointment in his repeated failures, he may lose confidence and stop trying altogether.

Harsh methods used to force a child to sit on the pot are self-defeating in most cases. Under excessive pressure, toilet habits may become a battleground between the child and his parents in which he will strongly resist in order to maintain his growing independence. Eventually a child will gain bowel control in spite of anxious pushings by his parents, but it will probably be later than he could have achieved it, and it may cause him to have concern about his bowels to an abnormal degree later on in life.

Lack of training is also self-defeating. When a child is left completely to his own devices, he may continue to wet and soil for a long time. Such freedom may be pleasurable to the child at the time, but he is denied the satisfaction that comes with real accomplishments.

Eventually our child no longer needs our assistance in developing toilet habits. Most children achieve bowel and bladder control because it pleases their parents. Our child's success is another indication he has taken an additional important step in the gradual acceptance of our values of living. Bowel and bladder control adds to a child's sense of achievement and sense of independence. He has gained confidence that will help him succeed in other aspects of the maturing process. The friendly teamwork between parent and child that went into the learning of toilet habits sets a pattern for other warm working relationships in the child's drive toward maturity. A healthy respect for the body gained at this time will lay the groundwork for the development of a healthy adult sexuality.

Oedipus Complex

The years from four to six witness an intensification of the sexual drive. The child develops an intense interest in his own body. What does it feel like? What is it for? Also he has great curiosity about the pleasures that he gets from deliberate manipulation of his genitals. Thus, masturbation is not an uncommon occurrence at this age. In general, most authorities agree that no harm is done by the child's discovery that his genital organs have pleasurable sensations surrounding them, as long as we adults don't make a big issue of it. Here again, we need to teach the child the correct behavior without making him feel ashamed about a natural feeling. We can say something such as this:

"I know it feels good to touch your penis. God made it that way. But little boys shouldn't sit on the pot all day, so get up and run out to play." The child's feelings have been acknowledged, but he is gently encouraged to find other interests. When a little girl discovers her clitoris and tells her mother that it is "her best feeling place," it takes a lot of love and faith not to say, "Don't touch." Actually, it is a reason for joy that the child has progressed normally so that her most pleasurable sensations no longer come from the mouth or anus, but from the genitals.

At this time, the preschooler often assumes that he can grow up and marry the parent of the opposite sex. The boy falls in love with his mother and the daughter is infatuated with her father. This early love triangle, called by Sigmund Freud the Oedipus Complex, was named after the Greek myth of Oedipus who slew his father and married his mother.

Not always openly expressed, such youthful fantasies are accompanied by all the ardor and tenderness at the child's command. But there remains the inconvenient complication that the parent already has a spouse. In his fantasy world, the child arranges solutions to this problem. He may say such things as, "Daddy can marry Grandma," or "Mommy can go next door." Jealousy of, and the wish to replace, the parental rival takes on many disguises. Proposing that she take her mother's place in bed with her father, a four-year-old girl then suggested that "Mommy can sleep on the floor."

The parent should not be frightened by the child's infatuation, but should understand that this is a normal part of growing up. We as parents can help the child through this period by sympathetically but firmly making clear in words and actions that the child cannot replace the rival parent and marriage must wait until he is older and can find a partner his own age.

When Gail announced that she was going to marry her father, her mother replied, "I know you like your father, but he and I are married. When you grow up, you will find someone you love very much to marry."

These passionate attachments of the preschooler come to grief when the girl realizes that she cannot compete with her mother for the affection of her father and the boy sees that he is no match for his father for his mother's affection. But in the process of going through this Oedipal period, the child grows in his own identity. The boy can strive to be as manly as his father and the girl as feminine as her mother. As the child enters the school years, the memories of this conflict are soon repressed. By the second grade, when a boy thinks that girls are sissy and dumb, he usually finds it unimaginable that he had once proposed taking his mother on a picnic and leaving daddy at home.

Sample Questions and Answers

This list of sample questions and answers is not intended to cover all of the questions that the small child will ask. They, along with questions discussed in the text, serve only as examples of the types of questions the preschooler may ask and suggest a way they can be answered in terms understandable to the child.

Where did I come from?

With this question, the child may be asking any of a number of things. Occasionally he may be asking a geographic question, really wanting to know from what city or town he came. Often he is seeking assurance that he belongs to the family and is really asking, "Who do I belong to?" He may be asking a spiritual or philosophical question. He may have heard that God made people and he is indeed trying to find out if this is so. Certainly many children who ask this question are wondering how they were made and have a vague idea about the truth. So, before we plunge into a long explanation of pregnancy and childbirth, it is best to ask the child, "What do you mean?" If it is apparent he is curious about his birth, we may begin the answer in this way:

"You grew in your mother's body. All mothers have a special place where babies grow."

How do babies get out?

"Mothers have a special opening between their legs that allows a baby to come out when he is ready."

*When a baby comes out, how can
you tell if it is a boy or a girl?*

"Boys and girls have different bodies. When a baby is born, it doesn't have any clothes on and the parents can tell if it is a boy or a girl by looking at its body."

How does a baby get inside the mother?

"The baby begins as a tiny egg. It gets food from the mother. After many months, the baby is big enough to be born."

Will I have a baby, too?

If a girl asks this question, we can answer, "Yes, when you grow up and get married."

If a boy asks, we may answer, "No, boys do not have a special place for babies to grow like girls. Boys will be fathers when they grow up."

Why do mothers have breasts?

"The breasts produce milk for the new baby. Only girls have breasts. Boys don't."

Questions For Discussion and Thought

1. To be loved is a primary need of infants. Without it they fail to grow mentally, physically and emotionally. In what ways do we as parents convey our love to our babies?

2. What names does your child use for penis, vagina, urinate, bowel movement? Will the names he uses now be appropriate for him to use when he is a teenager and an adult?

3. What kind of problems might result from toilet training that is too rigid? From too little training?

4. What might result if a child succeeds in his efforts to come between his parents and wins first place in the affection of his parents of the opposite sex?

Chapter 9

◆

The School Age Child:
Age Six to Eleven

What Is He Like?

The period of childhood, extending roughly from the time the child begins school to puberty, is a plateau. The rate of biologic growth lessens and a stable personality develops. Characteristically, the intensity of family ties is diluted by his world of friends, teachers, and other adults. Much of the curiosity formerly invested in babies and bottoms is now absorbed in mystery stories, secret clubs, codes, and batting averages of baseball heroes. Muscular coordination matures to where the child learns to ride a bike, bake a cake, dive, and pitch a no-hitter. Emotional control also stabilizes and the youngster is able to postpone gratification, control tears, and have fewer temper outbursts.

By the age of eight or nine, the previous attachments to home have decreased still more, and loyalty to school friends and the "gang" becomes more prominent. Affection plays only a small part at this time, and what affection there is is still directed toward the parents. The child is more interested in children of the same sex, and close friendships are often formed. Somewhat later a great admiration for an older person may develop, again usually for a person of the same sex. But in most instances the person admired remains unaware of the child's admiration since the child is shy and inarticulate about such things.

The child of this age is developing rapidly so far as his intellectual growth is concerned. His great thirst for knowledge is satisfied through school, reading, hobbies and clubs. His boundless energy can be rather easily channeled into worthwhile pursuits. He is very interested in the facts and often questions statements to make sure they are factual. But facts given in a straightforward manner are absorbed endlessly.

He wants to make and is able to make limited choices. Parents can profit by giving the school age child every opportunity to decide things for himself. Of course he is not ready or equipped to run his life without supervision but he can make decisions about what to wear, what to do with his free time, or what hobby he wants to pursue. This will build up his ego as well as give him experience for making much more difficult and important decisions later on.

What Is He Like Sexually?

The intense sexual curiosity of the preschool years and oedipal period is turned to other pursuits by the school age child. By and large, he is more interested in exploring his external environment and absorbing facts than he is in sexual matters. His sexual questions are fewer and more matter-of-fact. Modesty becomes important. He naturally wants to keep himself covered and is not nearly as interested in bare bodies and genitals as he once was or later will be.

This temporary lessening of sexual interest around six or seven years of age and extending over the grade school years was called "latency" by Sigmund Freud. Although psychologists and psychiatrists debate the meaning of latency and whether it exists or not, it is apparent that sexual interest does not disappear but only quiets down during this period.

The reason for this is not known. Some, including Freud, believed it to be an artefact of our puritanical society. In other words, as the child becomes more aware of the adult's disdainful view of sex, he unconsciously represses his own interests in the subject. Although this is probably a real factor, there seems to be more to the latency of sex interest at this age. For one thing, hormones are less active than they will be at puberty. Also intellectual pursuits absorb a large part of the child's energy at this age. Both boys and girls are more interested in why rockets fly, insects sting, and trees grow than they are in each other.

But sexual interests are not dormant, they are just toned down. While partly channeled into new interests and skills, they are also better concealed from adult eyes. Masturbation not only becomes less frequent but is more private. Reading permits independent investigations into dictionaries and home medical books for sexual information. Age mates become research partners in the game of "I'll show you mine if you will show me yours." Children become adept at telling sexually oriented jokes on the school ground and then blushing.

During this period boys stick with boys and girls with girls. A boy who prefers girl's activities is a sissy; to show an interest in one's mother is similarly disdained, except of course, in a moment of pain, sadness, and tender sentimentality. The taboos of associating with the opposite sex are less strong among girls; if invited, most will welcome inclusion in boy's activities; but being excluded, the girls generally band together in their contempt for the boy's rough and dirty play.

What Do They Want to Know About Sex?

The questions which children of school age want to have answered, whether they ask them or not, concern the origin of babies, the process of birth, the father's part in reproduction, the sex organs and their functions, and marriage. Great detail is unnecessary and often confusing. It is preferable to answer each question simply but adequately and then allow the child to ask another question.

By ten or eleven years of age many children who have not received adequate instruction become disturbed and worry about what the facts really are. They seek to remedy deficiencies in their knowledge by whispered conferences with their friends, by personal investigation and by reading books. Girls, particularly, may become resentful because of parental failure in this phase and may refuse to listen to any information which is offered. They may become moody and worried.

This can often be prevented by instruction during the early school years even if no, or few, questions have been asked. Giving a child a book from which to obtain sex information is certainly not adequate. Although all the necessary information may be included, it is frequently not suited to the particular child's needs and may not answer his specific questions.

Preadolescent girls should be instructed about menstruation, development of the breasts, and changes in the body shape. The girl of nine or ten is bound to hear whispered references to menstruation. If she does not have an understanding of the basic facts, she can become terribly confused by the piecemeal information that comes from her peers. Certainly, it is not unheard-of for the nine- or ten-year-old to begin menstruating; at least, they are likely to have friends who do.

The father can ordinarily discuss matters of sex with his son. The preadolescent boy should be prepared to expect the occasional emission of semen. He should understand that this, like the erection, is a natural occurrence, and that it is nature's way of taking care of sex activity until he is mature enough to assume the responsibility of marriage. The boy need not be disturbed by these occurrences if he leads a healthy, active life.

The child's relative evenness of emotions and his superior intellectual comprehension indicates that this is the optimal time at which to complete his enlightenment as to the major facts of reproduction. The youngster's greater comfort with the same sex suggests that the father can best teach the son and the mother, the daughter. Nevertheless, information and attitudes now come from many sources such as advertising, television, companions on the playground, as well as from teachers and parents.

Some parents delay preparing the child for puberty as if they might thus postpone the ferment of adolescence. The fact is, however, that the upheaval is likely to be greater in the face of ignorance. Parents should know that the glandular clock cannot be turned back. Some parents, never having experienced such preparation themselves, feel helpless to find the right word and welcome outside help in doing a better job than their own parents did.

How to Teach Them About Sex?

At this age, the learning process becomes more intentional than accidental. It is no longer just a by-product of experience and play. This, along with the child's preoccupation with facts, indicates that this is a good age at which to present much of the factual information about sex. While not having a morbid curiosity about sex, per se, the school age child will be quite interested in matter-of-fact explanations of how the body functions.

We must emphasize that explanations of facts or answers to questions need not be extremely detailed or involved. The amount of detail an answer requires will depend on many factors, but in general the seven-year-old will not need as complete an answer as the nine-year-old. The scope of sex interest, like the growth of appetites and heights, increases with years. The sex information a child requires cannot be administered in one single dose any more than can vitamin requirements.

For instance, the seven-year-old asking how the baby got into mommy's tummy doesn't have to have a detailed blow-by-blow description of sexual intercourse. However, he is ready for the basic facts such as "When mothers and fathers are ready to make a baby, the father puts his penis in the mother's vagina and releases sperm or seeds which fertilize the egg in the mother's uterus. The egg then grows into a baby over a period of nine months."

SAMPLE QUESTIONS AND ANSWERS

The following are some of the questions commonly asked by school-age children and they reflect the school-age child's preoccupation with factual information. This list is not intended to be complete but serves only as an example of the kind of questions and suggested answers.

Where was I before I was born?

"You were inside of your mother. You began as a tiny egg smaller than a grain of sand. Over nine months you grew until you were the size of a baby. When you were big enough to live outside, you were born."

Where do babies live before they are born?

"They live inside the mother. Each mother has a place called a uterus or womb that is a nesting place for babies. The baby lives and grows there until he is big enough to live outside. Then he is born."

Why do you need a doctor when the baby is born?

"The doctor helps the baby to be born. The doctor makes sure that both mother and the baby stay well and strong at this time."

How does the baby get outside of the mother?

"When the baby is large enough to live outside of his mother, the uterus or nest begins to grow smaller. This pushes the baby out of the mother through the birth canal or vagina."

Does the baby hurt the mother when he is born?

"The mother usually feels some pain when the baby is born but this is for only a little while. Mothers love their babies so much that they soon forget about the pain they might have had when he was born."

What is the navel for?

"When you were growing inside of your mother, there was a tube that connected you with your mother so that food could enter your body. That tube was attached to your body in your abdomen or belly. The navel is where the tube was attached."

What are breasts for?

"When the baby is growing inside of the mother, the breasts get ready to provide milk. After the baby is born the breasts produce milk that is perfect for the baby. Sometimes mother feeds the baby milk from the breast and sometimes from a bottle."

What does pregnant mean?

"When a woman is pregnant she is getting ready to have a baby. Pregnant means that a baby is growing inside of her. After the baby is born, she is no longer pregnant."

Are fathers necessary for babies to be made?

"Yes, mothers cannot make babies by themselves. When mothers and fathers get ready to have a baby, the father inserts his penis into the mother's vagina and deposits sperms that fertilize the egg in the mother's uterus. Then the egg begins to grow into a baby."

Questions For Discussion and Thought

1. "By school age the previous attachments to parents and family lessen as the child's loyalty and affection is diverted toward his peers." Do parents sometimes feel threatened by this? How can parents encourage this independence while at the same time maintaining a close relationship?

2. One of the common problems in the school age child is the picking up from peers and older children dirty words and obscene behavior. Suggest some good ways parents could react to an outburst of obscenity from an eight-year-old son.

3. What might be the emotional effect on a girl if she were to begin menstruation before she had been prepared by a proper explanation?

4. What problems would a boy growing up without a father have?

Chapter 10

◆

Adolescence: Introduction

Adolescence is difficult to define, but then a definition is hardly needed by anyone who has lived through it.

Adolescence can be described as an ill-defined period roughly paralleling the teenage years, spanning that part of a youth's life between childhood and adulthood during which he is neither an adult nor a child. The outstanding characteristic of adolescence is change: it is a period of rapid physical, sexual, personal, and intellectual growth.

The onset of adolescence is heralded by puberty, the earliest age at which a growing boy or girl becomes able to reproduce. Puberty, itself, is marked by the physical maturation of the sexual organs.

Physical Changes at Puberty

A sudden spurt in the linear growth (increase in length of the body, arms, and legs) is usually the first sign of puberty. This rapid acceleration of growth is due to the outpouring of sex and growth hormones into the blood stream from the thyroid, pituitary, and adrenal glands, and from the ovaries in girls and the testes in boys. It begins earlier in girls than in boys. Thus during the early stages of adolescence girls in general will be taller than boys of the same age. However, the female hormone, estrogen, soon slows the growth in girls at around age fourteen or fifteen while boys continue to grow. So around the midteen years, boys tower over their female peers and are still growing.

Soon after the growth spurt accelerates, the sex organs begin to mature. The internal and external sex organs of both male and female are well-developed but immature at birth. For example, the testes are essentially the same size at nine or ten years of age as they were when the boy was born. At puberty the genital organs begin to increase in size as well as in ability to function.

Due to hormones released by the growing genitals, secondary sexual characteristics begin to appear. Girls develop the feminine body contour, the boy's voice deepens, the girl's breasts begin to bud and grow and both boys and girls develop the characteristic male or female pattern of body hair growth. Finally, boys are able to produce sperm and ejaculate and girls to ovulate and menstruate. Their bodies are now ready for reproduction.

The age at which puberty begins is highly variable and is dependent on racial, climatical, emotional, nutritional, and cultural factors. Puberty occurs earlier in warmer than in colder climates. Poor nutrition delays the onset and certain cultural factors accelerate it. In general, girls begin puberty one to two years earlier than boys. The average age for the beginning of puberty in this country is 12½ years for girls and 13 to 14 years for boys.

Emotional Changes During Adolescence

Adolescence is a time of rapid physical, psychological and social changes. Most cultures, primitive and modern, recognize the significance of adolescence and provide an opportunity through rituals, games and initiation rites for the adolescent to find himself or herself and assure him or her of their place in the adult society. Whatever the culture, one of the challenges of this period involves the adolescent coming to grips with himself. "Who am I?", "Where am I going?", "What is my place in life?" are questions common to adolescents.

Normal adolescence has elements inevitably disturbing to adults. The adolescent must test and rebel against values, goals, and limits of his elders before he accepts some and rejects others. It is characteristic of adolescents that they vacillate from mature adult thinking one minute, or one day, to irresponsibility and childlike behavior the next.

In general, adolescents are defiant (to a greater or lesser extent) of parental authority, sharply critical toward prevailing social values and customs, committed deeply to religious and social belief (sometimes different from their parents), and they have strong attachments and loyalty to peer groups.

Two major developmental steps occur during adolescence: final dissolution of the direct dependence on the parents and the achievement of what Eric Erikson calls a "sense of identity." Both of these steps are critical to the health and happiness of the individual. A child who never gains financial, emotional, and social independence of his parents is in a real sense crippled and limited — he is not a mature person. Developing a sense of identity, a feeling of who he is and where he is going, is also a vital step toward maturity. The healthy turmoil of adolescence is a natural and necessary step in the metamorphosis of the child into the adult. Somewhere in the older teen years or early twenties, the adolescent emerges with the particular abilities and idiosyncrasies that he brings to his adult responsibilities of work, family and society at large.

The adolescent's move to the world of his contemporaries is accompanied by an emotional withdrawal from home and parents. Most parents are familiar with the "wall of silence" at the dinner table, the locked bedroom door, and the emphatic declarations that communication between the generations is no longer possible. Painful though it is for parents, the adolescent's noisy demands for an independent existence pave the way for mature adulthood.

By late adolescence, roughly the college years, rapid physical growth has ceased and the body has become more familiar and predictable. The adolescent is now more at home with himself and better able to control his emotions; impulsiveness and mercurial moodiness begin to wane. A variety of roles, values and interests will have been explored and commitment to some will have been made.

Preoccupation With Bodily Changes

After puberty, adolescents may not know why they feel different about their bodies, their behavior, and the opposite sex. They may not know about hormones and body change but they do know that they "feel" different. They are very self-conscious about their rapidly changing bodies and may wonder if they are normal. They often don't know that others their own age have the same doubts and anxieties.

Even when intellectually well prepared, most youngsters experience mixed feelings as a once familiar body changes almost daily. Budding breasts to the girl and bulging biceps to the boy may be welcomed, but pimples are not. Breast development may seem too much too soon or too little too late. The adolescent is constantly wondering what others think of his appearance. He is proud and yet uncertain about any bodily change that betrays his developing sexuality. While extremely proud of his enlarging penis, the boy is often acutely embarrassed when he finds that it produces a bulge in his bluejeans. A girl can hardly wait for her first bra, but then is horribly ashamed when a strap drops into sight. Simply standing before a group may produce anxiety because of fantasies about what others see in their bodies.

At times it is difficult for parents to understand a teenager's preoccupation with his body. But by under standing these real if somewhat exaggerated fantasies, the parents can do much to help the adolescent through this trying phase of his life.

Sexual Excitability

John, who was thirteen years of age, had come to my office complaining of an abdominal pain. After the exam revealed him to be quite healthy, I had asked if there was anything he wanted to talk to me about.

He hesitated at first and stared at the floor. "Well yes," he said anxiously. "I've been wondering if I'm normal or not — sex is always on my mind."

John summed up succinctly the sexual conflicts that grip the adolescent. The same hormones that are pro-ducing bodily changes are also stirring up sexual urges and thoughts that cannot be repressed. A glance or touch can excite, double meanings and innuendoes are read into the most casual remarks. The physical and emotional changes at puberty demand that each individ-ual come to terms with not only a changing body but with sexual conflicts and desires.

Heightened sexual excitability finds expression in ac-tion, feeling and thought. More quickly aroused, boys are quicker to discharge excitement through masturba-tion. Girls, who are more likely to suppress their mas-turbation, often seem to be in a state of perpetual day-dreams about some hoped-for "prince charming." In their fantasies, boys are more likely to dwell on specific bodily attributes — breasts, legs, and genitals while girls imagine romantic adventures of surrender. Some adoles-cents attempt to control sexual fantasies and impulses with a variety of maneuvers. For example, some put off homework so late that bedtime and exhaustion will overcome the temptation; others conscientiously count the number of days they have abstained. In all of this, the adolescent is struggling to gain control over the body that is powerful and mysterious.

A premature flight into intercourse is taken by some young people as a more normal or moral alternative to masturbation. Others may do so to test their desirability or to find acceptance that they are afraid they will not get otherwise. One young girl with a deformed arm chose "love without commitment" fearing that her deformity would keep boys from loving her for herself. Such motivations as these, along with group or parental pressure, may push a young adolescent into premature intercourse as a way of expressing his heightened sexuality.

The Christian adolescent experiences the same sexual impulses as others. These young people know that if some of their impulses were carried out, harm to themselves and others would be the result. They can't deny the feelings, yet they honestly want to do what is right. They are caught asking themselves, "Who is the real me?"

One fourteen-year-old boy asked during a group discussion of sex in a Sunday school class: "I dream about girls a lot — you know with their clothes off! Is that a sin? Is it adultery?" This young man was dedicated and earnest and more honest than most, yet he was expressing the feelings that grip him and most of his peers.

The Christian parent can do much to help the adolescent through this trying period. A basic understanding of the facts about sexual development gained during the preadolescent years will help the growing young person understand why he feels as he does. A warm open relationship between the parents and child during the preadolescent years will help the adolescent find the support he needs. On the other hand, the adolescent whose need for closeness has been frustrated in childhood, frequently grasps at sex now that it is available, and uses it to satisfy his unfulfilled need of belonging.

Openness between the adolescent and his parents will help get the feelings out into the open. If the adolescent knows that his parents understand and care, he will be more able to cope with his dilemmas. Also the adolescent who observes a happy and congenial sexual adjustment in his parents will probably see married life as something worth waiting for and find it easier to resist premature sexual experimentation.

However, the Christian adolescent is still a real person and cannot deny his sexuality. He will express his sexuality in many ways, through talk, fervent activity, competition and healthy dating. Also the Christian adolescent will experience some masturbation, nightly emissions, and sexual fantasies. The parent of the adolescent should not become concerned about this or feel that the adolescent is condemned for these normal signs of growing up.

Sexual Identity

The first struggle for sexual identity occurs during the preschool years when the child begins gradually but assuredly to take on the characteristics of male or female. It reaches its peak in the conflicts of the Oedipal period and then quiets down during the grade school years when the child is absorbed in peer group activities.

The rapid changes of adolescence reawaken uncertainties about sexual identity. During the grade school years, the adolescent has been primarily interested in peers of the same sex. Now at adolescence he is caught up in strong sexual attractions but is unsure how to relate to the opposite sex. At this time in life young people are suddenly unsure of their own masculinity or femininity. They see things in themselves that they think contradict their sex role. The boy may religiously exercise to develop large biceps to prove his masculinity or may engage in dangerous or questionable acts to "prove" his bravery as well as his maleness. The budding adolescent girl may use excessive make-up or wear provocative clothes to prove herself femininely attactive. Occasionally, particularly in the presence of ignorance about the real meaning of sex, young adolescents may experiment with heavy petting and sexual intercourse to "prove" their potency or attractiveness.

The admiration which the preadolescent may feel for an older person may develop into a crush at adolescence. Usually, affection is centered on a person of the same sex. Often at this age fondness for some member of the same sex may vie with fondness for one of the other sex. Such a crush, or temporary fascination between two people of the same sex, is most often seen with adolescent girls, but occasionally it is seen between boys. Frequently an older person such as a teacher or entertainer is the object of such exaggerated admiration. Crushes usually have little erotic significance and run a brief course without dire consequences. But crushes are objectionable and should be discouraged since they lead to exclusion of friendships with other young people. Crushes should be handled with sympathy and understanding but the parent should encourage the child to develop a wide range of friendship.

While the teenager is embroiled in the search for sexual identity, he often has some brief, but frank homosexual thoughts. Often the adolescent wonders if he is a homosexual because of his contradictory thoughts. However, homosexuality is not produced by this natural search for sexual identity but is due to emotional disturbances produced early in life.

Parents can best help their teenagers through this struggle for sexual identity by being good models themselves. Girls develop their final concept of femininity by observing their mother, and boys model their masculinity after their father. Ideally, a relationship between mother and daughter and father and son will have developed during the childhood years. Though tested by adolescent independence, it will continue to exist. As mother and daughter share confidences and father and son talk "men talk" the adolescent will gain confidence in his role as a sexual creature.

Confusion of Love and Sex

Adolescents often confuse "love" with "sex." The adolescent is bombarded with this confused concept of sexuality from every media — TV, movies, books, and advertisements. Such song titles as "Love Me Tonight"; "Why Don't We Do It in the Road," and "Gimme, Gimme, What You've Got," only add to the adolescent's confusion on this point.

A group of thirteen- and fourteen-year-old girls, pregnant out of wedlock, stated that records and TV, particularly soap operas with the heavy dose of adultery and illicit sex, turned them on sexually. The heavy emphasis on "Making Love" in our society is misleading to the adolescent who does not yet have the factual or emotional maturity to see that love is much more than something you do in the backseat at a drive-in movie.

Of course, the witnessing of a true love relationship between parents will go a long way in helping adolescents put love and sex in its proper perspective. In addition, helping them to become familiar with books, plays and movies that show love and sex in their proper relationship will help counteract the heavy dose of illicit sex that saturates our society. Needless to say, the adolescent involved in religious training and activities will more likely assign sex a proper place in his life.

Dealing With the Adolescent's Budding Sexuality

Several suggestions have already been made as to how parents can respond to the adolescent's surge of sexual interest. In this section we will pull together some additional ideas on coping with what to some parents is a most exasperating part of their child's plunge toward maturity.

First of all, the parent should not be shocked or dismayed by adolescents' relative preoccupation with sex. It is quite normal. As a matter-of-fact, the adolescent who does not seem interested in sex is the one who is likely to have problems. Such young people are experiencing the same hormonal pressures as the others, they just keep their conflicts inside. But sooner or later they are likely to explode either into a neurotic illness that will likely be lifelong, or they may become easy prey to sexual exploitation by the unscrupulous. As often as not, it is the wallflower, theoretically not interested in sex, who gets pregnant out of wedlock; or the quiet boy who never showed any interest in girls who easily falls prey to homosexual overtures.

So parents should accept their child's interest in sex as a healthy development. This does not imply that the adolescent should be given license for any and all behavior. But his curiosity can be accepted as normal and healthy.

The key to success is keeping the lines of communication open: let the adolescent know you understand and sympathize with his conflicts while at the same time letting him know exactly what you feel is proper and improper sexual behavior.

Parents should try to understand the sex needs of the adolescent. A cheerful, interested, but not obviously watchful, attitude will help the young person through his periods of uncertainty. To ridicule early infatuations, or make the adolescent feel guilty about something he has said or written forfeits his confidence and precludes the possibility of communicating with him.

Adolescence is a trying time for both parents and offspring. But if both parents and adolescents "hang in there" it can be the most rewarding years of parenthood, for out of adolescence comes the product of all the parent-child interactions — a mature adult.

This chapter has discussed in general terms some of the characteristics and problems of adolescence. Adolescent boys and girls share many of the same problems and questions but they also have many unique to their sex. The next two chapters will discuss adolescent sexuality as it applies to girls and boys separately.

Questions For Discussion and Thought

1. What about adolescence is most disturbing to adults?
2. How can parents help their adolescents develop a healthy sense of identity: i.e., to really know who and what they are?
3. How can parents help their teenager deal with his real and often exaggerated fantasies about his body?
4. How can parents help their teenagers develop a proper sexual identity?

Chapter 11

◆

The Adolescent Girl

"Do you think a girl should wave at boys she doesn't know when she passes them on the street?"

"If you had a daughter our age, would you allow her to go steady?"

"Say a girl really likes a boy and something happens to him, like he gets killed — is it wrong for her to think about him?"

"Does a girl produce an egg sort of half way through her menstrual cycle?"

"What happens during a miscarriage?"

"How can a woman get pregnant by just sleeping with a man?"

"If a boy and girl are going to get married, is it all right for them to have intercourse?"

"Does it embarrass you to answer these questions?"

These are just a few of the questions asked by thirteen- and fourteen-year-old girls during a group discussion of sexual questions led by a perceptive Sunday school teacher. These questions illustrate the intense concern adolescent girls have about sex. They also dramatically illustrate the varied interests of teenage girls. Their interests include a real concern about the etiquette of boy-girl relationships, a determined search for the facts of menstruation, pregnancy and intercourse, and an honest concern for what it right and wrong.

*Helping the Adolescent Girl Under-
stand Physical Changes at Puberty*

Starting somewhere between the seventh and tenth year, an area deep in the brain, called the hypothalmus, stimulates the pituitary gland to secrete a variety of hormones. One of these hormones, in turn, stimulates the immature ovary to produce the female hormone, estrogen. Estrogen then causes growth of the pelvis and deposition of fat in the breasts and hips producing the typical female figure. Estrogen also causes growth of the nipples and budding of the mammary glands so that the breasts begin to fill out, giving the girl a definite sign of her womanhood. The external genitalia, including the clitoris and the labia, begin to enlarge in response to estrogen. The internal genitalia also mature. The vagina enlarges and begins to produce mucous. The uterus enlarges and the special lining called the endometrium begins to form.

Somewhere between the age of ten and eighteen years, an event of great magnitude occurs in the life of every girl: She begins to menstruate. The average age of menarche, the medical term for the beginning of menstruation, is twelve to thirteen years of age. But menarche may occur as early as nine or ten or as late as fifteen to sixteen in perfectly normal girls. The timing of menarche is determined by many factors, but the single most important one is heredity. A girl's menstrual pattern will likely follow that of her mother. If her mother started early, around ten or eleven, the daughter is likely to start early. If her mother was fifteen or sixteen before her menses started, then the daughter is likely to be normally late also.

Many girls, as well as their mothers, become concerned when they do not start their periods at eleven or twelve as many of their peers do. Such a girl is likely to be completely normal, but if she or her family is worried she should see her family physician. Probably, he can assure all concerned that she is healthy and normal.

Since some girls experience menarche as early as nine or ten or, if not, they will have friends who do, it is quite important to educate the preadolescent in the fact of, and facts about menstruation. If this information is delayed and menses starts before the girl is prepared, severe psychological problems may arise.

Early adolescent girls are emotionally and intellectually ready for a complete and detailed explanation of reproductive physiology. The parents should be ready to discuss these facts but girls will also benefit by a presentation of anatomy and physiology at school or church. Group discussions of common concerns is often an effective way to relay information during early adolescence. To be complete, the girl's education should include a discussion of male as well as female anatomy and physiology. Girls are naturally curious about the opposite sex. If their curiosity is satisfied through instruction, illicit experimentation will be less likely.

Questions About Menstruation

The following questions about menstruation certainly do not cover the whole subject, but they are intended as examples of the type of questions girls ask and how they can be answered.

1. Just what is the menstrual period?

"The menstrual period is a symbol of womanhood. It is a sign that your body is preparing for your role as a mother when you get married. Each month the uterus, or womb, prepares a fresh nesting place for a tiny egg. If the egg is not fertilized, the nest is shed in the form of a bloody fluid which makes up the menstrual flow."

2. Are variations in the menstrual cycle normal?

"Yes, the length of the menstrual cycle varies from girl to girl. Periods are usually anywhere from twenty to thirty-five days apart. The menstrual period itself varies from three to six days but in most girls it will be four or five days. At first a girl's cycle may be quite irregular. For example, it may be twenty-three days one month, thirty the next. But after a few months most girls fall into a regular dependable pattern."

3. Should I use a pad or a tampon?

"The answer to this question depends on several factors but for the most part a girl can use either. It is a common misconception that a virgin cannot wear a tampon but this is not true. Most can wear them very comfortably. The choice between tampons or pads depends on the personal preference of mother and daughter. If in doubt consult your personal physician about what is best."

4. Should I go on a date when I am having a period?

"With a proper understanding of menstruation and knowledge of hygiene girls need not change or regulate their social life to fit their menstrual periods. With proper protection you should be able to enjoy activities that you normally participate in without fear. There is no need for your date, or anyone else, to be aware of your period. Certainly as a precaution, a girl should always carry extra napkins or tampons in her purse."

Other Questions Adolescent Girls Ask

1. What's wrong with a girl calling a boy on the telephone?

All adolescent girls are preoccupied with boys. They think, talk and dream boys. Particularly in early adolescence, the girls are more interested in boys than boys are in girls. Most girls are interested in the proper etiquette of boy-girl relationships, but they often need guidance in understanding what is appropriate. A suggested answer to the question is the following:

"A girl should not call a boy because he might get the idea she is chasing him. Certainly, this is the last thing that you want him to think, particularly if you really are chasing him. The quickest way to turn off a boy is to let him know that you are after him."

2. Who has a stronger sex drive, girls or boys?

"While both males and females have sex drives that are equally strong, boys are more easily aroused than girls. Heavy petting, such as genital manipulation, arouses boys to a very high intensity. Unfortunately the responsibility for enforcing restraint will almost always rest with the girl."

3. Why can't I date an older person?

Since girls often begin puberty before boys of their age, they are sometimes attracted to, and attract, boys or men several years their senior. Parents should try to help their daughter understand that it is best for her to become acquainted with boys her own age since their interests are more in common. Also the parent needs to explain that the intentions of older boys or men are often less than ideal.

4. How do you know you are going to have a baby?

"The mother realizes it first when she misses a menstrual period. A checkup with her doctor can confirm the presence of pregnancy."

5. Do unmarried people get pregnant?

"Yes, an adult woman can get pregnant whether she is married or not if she has intercourse. In fact, thousands of babies are born each year without a real home because their parents had intercourse outside of marriage. Such pregnancies are usually tragic. We, as Christians, believe that intercourse, pregnancy and child rearing are for husband and wife only."

6. If a husband and wife don't want to have a baby, why do they have intercourse?

"Sexual intercourse is a gift of God to men and women. It not only serves as a means of procreation but also as a means of expressing love. A husband and wife have intercourse often as a way of relieving sexual tensions and as a means of showing their love for one another."

7. Is sexual intercourse painful?

"It should not be. It is painful only when one partner forces himself on the other or when one partner is not psychologically prepared for intercourse."

8. Is having a baby painful?

"Yes, a certain amount of pain is associated with childbirth. But there are psychological and medical means to lessen the pain and it is not as great as you might think. Certainly after the birth of the child, the pain is insignificant compared with the joy of holding the new baby."

9. Does a baby start every time you mate?

"No, only at certain times during the menstrual cycle (approximately halfway between periods) is the egg ripe for fertilization. For a baby to start its growth, the sperm must reach the egg at the right time and fertilize it."

10. What is a miscarriage?

"A miscarriage, or an abortion, is the termination of a pregnancy before the fetus is mature enough to live outside the mother. A miscarriage can be caused by several factors, including illness or accidents to the mother. The most common cause of a miscarriage is a defective egg or sperm."

Some Questions Parents Ask

1. My daughter is maturing early, how can I handle this?

There is great pressure in our society for teenagers to grow up too fast. In many communities, preteens are rushed into unchaperoned parties, dating and premature interests in sexual expression. Some parents actually encourage this, feeling that their daughter's "adult like" appearance is an asset to the family. Such a trend is dangerous. In spite of her physical appearance, the "well developed" twelve-year-old is still a twelve-year-old emotionally.

Parents of "early maturing" girls should encourage sensible clothing that flatters, but not "ages," the teenager. They should discourage the use of high heels, lipstick, and padded bras during the preteen years. Dress and play clothes (swim suits, etc.) should be stylish but moderate. Girls should be encouraged to participate in activities with her age peers of both sexes. Although she can be proud of her developing body, she should be encouraged to see life in perspective. She needs help in realizing that school, hobbies and friends are fun, as well as important.

2. My daughter doesn't show any interest in boys. Is this normal?

It very well may be. Some girls become interested in boys earlier than others. Girls who are late in physical development may be slow in becoming preoccupied with boys. If she continues to have friendships with both sexes and participates in school, church and peer group activities the parent can relax. She is probably normal. However, if she is not only withdrawn from boys but from most activities and becomes a recluse, she may be worried, shy or afraid. She may be embarrassed about her appearance or worried about whether she is able to control her impulses. In this case parents should try to find out what the problem is and get professional help from pastor, family physician or school counselor if it is needed.

3. Who should talk to the adolescent girl about sex? The mother or father?

The mother is the natural one to talk to her daughter about menstruation — after all she can speak from experience. In other matters, the mother can answer most of the girl's questions better than anyone else. The daughter is fortunate if her mother is open to her questions and shows an understanding of her feelings. Such a confidant can help her through many of the difficult emotional crises of an adolescent girl's life.

However, a girl's father can also be a real asset. He can serve as a strong shoulder to cry on when things aren't going well. He can help her understand how boys think and feel, and he can help her see the things boys appreciate in girls. As a male, he can help her budding self image by praising her assets and diplomatically helping her make improvements where they are needed. Along with the mother, he can set rules for the daughter's conduct and carefully explain that they are for her protection.

4. Should we tell our daughter about the sordid things?

Yes. She will hear about illegitimacy, pregnancy, dope, abortions and homosexuality from other sources. She will be better off if she feels free to discuss these things with her parents.

5. How can we be sure that our daughter will not get pregnant before marriage?

One way is to provide her with contraceptives and teach her how to use them. However, statistics show that contraceptives are not very effective with teenagers. In the heat of emotional sex play, most forget to use them. Besides, Christian parents rebel against this idea. Christian parents are not just interested in preventing out-of-wedlock pregnancy, but are interested in helping their daughter have a full abundant life, and they know that premature sexual commitment contradicts the goal, whether or not it results in pregnancy.

Parents can best insure that their daughter will remain chaste by doing these things:

1. Give their daughter a happy loving home with sexually satisfied parents.

2. Through teaching at home and at church, impress upon her, not a negative morality that is centered in "don'ts," but teach her a morality based on the worth of each individual and on each individual's responsibility to God.

3. Give her a thorough and appropriate sex education that satisfies her curiosity about the facts as well as gives her a positive concept of sexuality.

Questions For Discussion and Thought

1. "Does it embarrass you to answer these questions?" the teenage girl asked her Sunday school teacher. Would answering such questions embarrass you? How might you overcome such embarrassment?

2. Why should a girl have a full explanation of male sexual anatomy?

3. What can a father contribute to a girl's sex education?

4. How can parents reduce the pressure on teen girls to mature early?

Chapter 12

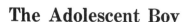

The Adolescent Boy

Adolescent boys are known for their boundless energy which they express in competitive sports, intellectual pursuits and, as often as not, making pests of themselves.

Although puberty starts later in boys than in girls, once it begins, the boy is just as overwhelmed with the sex drive as girls. Bob, who had just turned fourteen said, "I have these funny feelings when I see a girl — particularly a pretty girl. Later I feel guilty and wonder if it is normal to have these feelings."

When asked exactly what kind of feelings, he had said, "Well, I wonder what she looks like with her clothes off."

No doubt, adolescent boys are sexual creatures and need help in understanding and coping with the conflicting emotions that grip them.

Helping the Adolescent Boy Understand the Physical Changes of Puberty

As with girls, the age at which puberty begins is variable with boys. An increase in the size of the penis and testes is the first signal that puberty is beginning. Until puberty, the penis has grown little, and the testes almost none, since infancy. As the testes increase in size, they become quite sensitive to pressure. In the average boy these changes occur around thirteen years of age, but they may occur as early as ten or eleven or as late as fourteen to fifteen years. Shortly after these changes appear, the adolescent boy experiences a rapid spurt of growth that sends him towering above the girls of the same age, who up to now have been embarrassingly taller than he.

Some hair growth in the pubic region usually accompanies the increase in the size of the genitalia. During the growth spurt, this hair growth accelerates and takes on the male distribution. The appearance of hair on the chest, under the arms, and on the face is not as predictable. While some boys develop body hair and beard early in adolescence, others do not acquire these status symbols until late in the teenage years. The best prediction as to when the beard will appear is the age at which the boy's father began shaving. If the father began early, the son is likely to have a beard early; if the father was late his son will probably be so. The boy who is anxious about his lack of beard can be assured that he definitely will have one sooner or later. Suggest that he relax meanwhile, and enjoy his freedom from the razor.

Voice changes are characteristic of the adolescent boy and usually occur along with the growth spurt. The deepening of the voice to a more masculine tone is produced by growth of the larnyx or voice box. As the voice deepens, a prominent bump appears in the neck giving the boy his "Adam's apple." These voice changes are troublesome for some boys because the quality and tone of their voice is uncertain and undependable. As the growth spurt reaches its peak and levels off, the young man will have a stable voice with a deeper pitch.

Midway through puberty some boys experience enlargement of the breasts. Sometimes just one, sometimes both breasts are enlarged. This enlargement of the male breasts, called gynecomastia, is not only normal, but also temporary. It may last for eight to twelve months; rarely will it last longer. About half of adolescent boys experience gynecomastia to some degree. Coming at a time when he is acutely concerned about his masculinity, this can be embarrassing and threatening. Those who have gynecomastia often feel that they are less of a man because of it and they are frequently ridiculed by others. It is important to make clear to the boy that the breast enlargement is temporary, normal, and in no way threatens his masculinity. It may be mentioned that some of the strongest athletes have experienced this same problem.

As many parents have noticed, the penis is capable of an erection at birth. Infants and young boys may have erections when the genitalia are stimulated by cold, pressure, or friction. This is entirely normal and is no reason for concern. At puberty, boys become capable of an erection when stimulated emotionally. This, of course, is a natural prerequisite to adult sexual function and should be accepted by parents and boys alike as a healthy development.

There is no accurate data as to when the first ejaculation of semen occurs. However, the potential for ejaculation develops during the time that the boy's height and genitalia are rapidly growing. This is a milestone in the boy's life, in that the ability to produce sperm and ejaculate semen heralds the onset of his ability to reproduce. As the ability to ejaculate develops, the boy is likely to begin to have "wet dreams" or "nightly emissions." The boy may become concerned about this and needs assurance that he is normal.

Questions Boys Ask

Although not comprehensive, these questions will serve to illustrate what adolescent boys are thinking about.

1. What is a wet dream or nocturnal emission?

"This is a discharge of semen during sleep. Semen is produced and stored in little sacs near the bladder.

Periodically, there is a need for this semen to be discharged. Wet dreams are not a sign of disease or abnormal development. These do not indicate that a boy is 'oversexed,' nor can they cause any harm. In other words, they are completely normal."

2. What is a circumcision?

"Circumcision is a minor operation during which a portion of the foreskin of the penis is removed. It is usually done during the newborn period. It is sometimes done for medical reasons and sometimes for religious reasons."

3. Does the amount of hair on my chest have anything to do with how "manly" I am?

"No. The amount of body hair is determined by heredity and has no relationship to one's strength or ability to perform intercourse."

4. Sometimes my penis gets hard when I see a pretty girl. Is that normal?

"This is called an erection and you'll experience these often, either when your genitals are manipulated or when you are emotionally excited. The erection itself is normal and does not mean that you are morbid, oversexed or sinful. It is not sinful to think of girls in sexual terms — as long as you don't dwell on these thoughts and let them take over your life. The attraction between boys and girls is God-given. As long as boys are attracted to girls as individuals who have a soul and a mind as well as body, this attraction is healthy. Only when boys are attracted to girls as sexual creatures and nothing else is it wrong."

5. My penis is smaller than other boys'. Am I abnormal?

"There is a wide variation in the size of the external

genitals, just as there is variation in the size of the nose, ears, and fingers. The size of the penis has nothing to do with one's sexual attraction or potency."

6. What is menstruation?

Parents often ask if they should tell their teenage boy about menstruation. By all means, boys should be told. They will see advertisements for sanitary supplies and likely will see napkins around the house. Boys sooner or later notice that girls act differently at different times of the month. From other boys they will hear talk about menstruation, most of which is fantasy and misinformation. By helping him understand this aspect of female make-up not only will his curiosity be satisfied, but he will be able to understand and tolerate the woman's role more sensitively.

7. What is prostitution?

"Prostitution is the giving of one's body or sexual favors for hire. As commonly practiced, a woman will offer herself for sexual intercourse to any and all men who will pay the price. The women involved often work alone as 'streetwalkers' or work out of brothels or 'houses of prostitution' which are run by 'pimps' or 'producers.' Such women are frequently called 'prostitutes,' 'whores,' or 'harlots.'

"Prostitutes are patronized by men of high and low social status, by healthy and diseased men, by 'straight' and perverted ones. Thus prostitutes serve as an important source of venereal disease and one gets involved with a prostitute at his own risk."

8. What is homosexuality?

"Homosexuality is sexual attraction to, or sexual activity with, members of the same sex." (See Chapter 14 for more details.)

9. What does "jacking off" mean?

"This is a more or less vulgar term that some mis-informed people use when they are talking about mas-turbation. It is not a particularly polite term and I would prefer you to use 'masturbate' since it is the cor-rect term."

Questions For Discussion and Thought

1. How can parents help reassure the doubting adolescent boy that his masculinity is real and secure?
2. Is it best to let the teenage boy talk about his sexual feelings or to try to switch his attention to something else?
3. What part can his mother play in a teen boy's sex education?
4. What kind of false rumors did you hear about men-struation before you knew the truth? Do you think your son has heard the same rumors?

Chapter 13

Dating

Introduction

Barbara Wilson wanted to laugh and cry but she dared not do either. She was supposed to be the calm, assured mother. Assisting Sandra, her fifteen-year-old daughter, as she prepared for her first real date was really an emotional affair. Since Brian had called to ask her to the high school football game, Sandra's life had been in a whirl. Her immaculate attention to detail and her constant peeks in the mirror were really funny; but the tensions that burst within her were real.

Barbara could remember her own first date very well. The fear that gripped her then was fresh in her mind. She knew the thoughts that were racing through Sandra's mind: "What will I say?"; "What will we do?"; "What if I spill hot chocolate on my dress — Oh, I'll just die!"

To the American teenager, dating is the most significant event in his or her teenage years. It is of such importance to some, that life and death hang on getting a date with the right person. This privilege of dating, taken for granted by the American teenager, is a product of our western culture. In most of the Asian and African cultures, a word for dating does not exist in the language simply because dating does not exist. In these cultures, the activities of young people are closely supervised and family oriented. When they reach marriageable age, a marriage is arranged by the parents and the young people have little to say in the matter.

In these cultures, the system seems to work quite well. Often in such arranged marriages, the husband and wife fall genuinely in love. In fact, their divorce rate is much less than ours. Is it possible that the parents have more insight into the type of person that will make an appropriate mate for their child than the child does himself?

In recent times, the western system of mate selection has begun to influence these other cultures. We will have to wait and see if these "democratic changes" will be for the best.

Many American parents might wish for an opportunity to have more control over the mating selection process of their children. But this is not likely since dating is firmly fixed in our culture. Thus, parents should have some understanding of the dating system.

The Dating System

Dating as we know it is a modern development. Its intent may be casual or serious. Frequently the frivolous and the more serious intentions are intertwined. The dating system is a competitive, elaborate process that is youth-centered rather than parent-controlled. For better or worse, the system is flexible, democratic and romantic.

Studies have shown that dating in most communities is a process of sequential involvement as follows:

1. Group dating.
2. Random dating.
3. Casual going steady.
4. Serious going steady.
5. Informal engagement.
6. Formal engagement.

Of course, every teenager will not go through these steps in exactly the same manner or sequence. This outline represents the general trend.

During the past generation a significant revolution in the system has been "dating for dating's sake." Most dating today is nonmarriage oriented; the young people associate together simply for the fun of it. The specific purpose of a date depends on the individual. It may be for prestige, recreation, to make friends or for sexual excitement. This is in contrast to the past when dating, or courtship as it was then known, was serious in its direct focus on marriage.

What Age Is the Right Age?

Without doubt, there is a trend toward earlier and earlier dating. In some areas dating among junior high students, and in some cases, group dating among elementary school children, is not unusual. Parties and other functions are arranged so that these young students are encouraged to pair off. Girls whose breasts are hardly budding are dressed up in stockings and padded bras and both boys and girls are encouraged to have a boy friend or a girl friend. Teachers and eager mothers are frequently scheming to get Tom out of his baseball uniform and into his party clothes; he is scorned for not having a "proper" interest in girls. Often a pattern develops in a community in which everyone dates. The pressure is then on both parents and child to conform.

Many authorities believe that such early dating under pressure arouses resentment in many boys and girls who are not ready for dating. Other more serious dangers of premature dating exist. When boys and girls are forced to think of each other as sexual beings, sexual urges are excited way beyond normal. This presents an impossible conflict to preteens and early teenagers. A vicious cycle is set up in which more and more sexual excitement is sought for their frustrated drives. By the early teenage years this sexual excitement may be so great that the teenager can no longer resist and sexual intimacy becomes the next step. Early adolescents or preteens are too emotionally immature to cope with this and they can be psychologically harmed. One mother who started her "mature" twelve-year-old dating could not understand why the girl was pregnant before she was fourteen.

Well, when is the right time to let a teenager start dating? This is a question without any one answer. It depends on the personality and maturity of the teenager, the community customs and, most importantly, the family standards. But some general principles can be discussed.

In the older junior high school ages, approximately thirteen and fourteen years old, well supervised group dating may be appropriate. Well planned activities in which boys and girls mix and play together will allow each sex to get used to each other in a low pressure situation. While at these ages some pairing off occurs, it should not be encouraged. The important goal at this age is for the young people to get to know a variety of other people and to learn how to act, talk, and play with the opposite sex. Most authorities agree that single dating during the preteen or early teens is treacherous.

The parent of each child is in the best position to determine when that child is ready to single or double date alone. The wise parent will make this decision based on the maturity and personality of the child, the places and events available for dates, and community customs. The wise parent will resist pressures to put the child on his or her own too soon, but at the same time he will not restrict the growing adolescent too long. The boy or girl who is prevented from dating after he or she is ready will grow resentful and likely rebel. Somewhere in the early high school years, most boys and girls will want to, and probably should be allowed to, have dates to school affairs such as sport events, parties, and plays. Dates to non-school related events will be allowed as the parents see fit. In the early high school years, parents will have to carefully, but diplomatically, set limits on dating behavior, (where to go, when to get home, frequency of dates, etc.). Later in the senior year and the college years the parents may still set limits but these will be more relaxed. If sex education has been successful, young people of this age should be maturing and capable of making wise decisions for themselves.

Going Steady

Going steady, or limiting one's dating to one partner, is a modern revolution in dating and is quite common during the teen years. In some communities there is pressure even for the junior high students to go steady. In one study, seventy-seven percent of college students surveyed had gone steady with at least one person. In this study, random dating was the characteristic of ninth and tenth grades, while going steady was the primary pattern in the eleventh and twelfth grades.

There is evidence for two types of going steady in high school. One type is engaged in most by those intending to go to college and is essentially a "convenience relationship" which is not expected to result in marriage. It is a temporary arrangement of convenience. The other type is enjoyed by the non-college groups and is a more serious arrangement that is likely to lead to marriage.

Why do young people go steady?

In many communities it is a status symbol to have "a girl" or a "steady." If you don't have such a partner something must be wrong with you. Another reason is that it is social insurance — you don't have to worry about a date; you have an automatic date to all events. This arrangement is often attractive to girls who always worry about getting asked and for boys who are shy about calling girls whom they do not know well. A few insecure young people look on going steady as a way of finding security and love that they have not received at home. Their own self image is propped up by knowing that someone "likes" them well enough to go steady.

Authorities do not completely agree on whether going steady is good or bad. Some say that the steady relationship is less exploitative than random dating. In random dating one has the opportunity to use the partner, since the relationship is fleeting and one does not stick around to face the consequences. The reasoning goes that one is less likely to exploit someone he sees on every date and must repeatedly face in the light of day. However, others feel that going steady among early teens has more negative than positive values. Particularly in the early teen years, there is a need for boys and girls to meet a large number of peers and learn how to get along with a variety of people. Going steady necessarily limits flexibility in socializing. Also going steady too early may lead to boredom and, thus, sexual experimentation.

Again family standards and local customs will help parents decide whether their child should go steady. But in general, this practice should be discouraged until the later teen years.

Mate Selection

For some young people the senior year in high school is a time when they seriously begin to look for a suitable mate. Others begin their search in the college years. Dating becomes the prime instrument in selecting a marriage partner. The general process is that a dating couple find they have a lot in common and like each other's company. This leads to "falling in love," a state that is often highly emotional. This romantic love either leads to a more mature, deepening love or soon dies as the couple find that they were not made for each other after all. Danger exists when young people in their early teens "fall in love." At this age they are still too immature to really judge what love is. If such early romances result in a teenage marriage, the chance for a successful marriage is compromised. While a certain amount of puppy love is normal for young teens, wise parents will discourage serious romances at these ages.

Eventually, though, there comes a time when serious attention to mate selection is appropriate. Young people need criteria by which they can make wise choices at this point. Their expectations of marriage and of the marriage partner will largely reflect what they have witnessed in their own home. If they come from a happy home which cherishes high ideals, they will probably judge a potential mate by such personal qualities. If they come from a family where members are exploited by each other, they may very well select a mate whom they can easily exploit, or be exploited by. If they come from a family where prestige, fame, wealth, physical prowess is looked upon as the highest values, then the young person may select a mate who can provide these regardless of whether he or she has the personal qualities necessary for a congenial relationship. Parents need to help the teenager see the qualities which make a good mate so that the young person will be guided by more reliable criteria than just his or her emotions.

How Parents Can Help

Parents should make their rules about dating clear and unambiguous. The teenager should be given an explanation for the rules. Most teenagers realize that their parents are putting their welfare first and most will be reasonable in their demands if they see that their parents are reasonable. But parents must be on their guard lest they yield to the demand that "everyone is doing it."

At the same time parents can understand that adolescence is a trying time for boy or girl. Not being invited to the homecoming game can be a life and death matter. While they cannot solve the teenager's dating problem, parents can understand and provide a shoulder to cry on in crises.

The question arises, "Should I regulate whom my son or daughter dates?" While parents do not want their son or daughter dating just anyone, it is difficult for parents in our mobile society to scrutinize all of their children's friends. The best way to encourage your young people to have wholesome friends is early to instill in them high standards of personal conduct. Also by providing activities through church and school and by encouraging the young people to bring their friends home, parents can help them develop appropriate relationships.

Questions For Discussion and Thought

1. How old were you when you started dating? Would you like your child to start at the same age?
2. How can we as parents reduce the pressures for earlier and earlier dating on our children?
3. What do you think is the right age for girls to start dating in your community? For boys?
4. Your child is sixteen years old and wants to date but does not have any offers. How can you as a parent help in this situation?

Chapter 14

◆

Approaching Adulthood

As the conflicts of early adolescence resolve, the older teenager begins to find himself and his place in life. While still propelled by strong sexual emotions, he becomes more serious and intellectual about sex as well as other issues. His questions are penetrating and deep; he is not satisfied with superficial answers. As he completes high school and prepares for college or a full-time job, he should have successfully arrived at an independent personality. He is able to make decisions for himself and is no longer under direct control of his parents. But the training of his early years will not be lost. The goal of parenthood is a mature adult. Hopefully, the older teenager will have learned inner self-control; less and less external control from the parents will be required.

This chapter deals with several topics that are of great concern to the maturing teenager as well as his parents. Certainly, interest in these particular topics is not limited to the older teenager. Often young teenagers or preadolescents have questions about homosexuality, abortion, petting, etc. When questions are asked, they should be answered in language that is understandable to that particular child.

All the Way, Why Not?

General agreement exists that premarital sexual relations among high school and college students are more frequent than they were a generation ago. In our increasingly sexually permissive society, premarital coitus is becoming not only more possible, but, on the surface, more inviting to the teenager. Popular songs beg, "Let's Do It in the Road" or lament, "Why Not Tonight?"; these lyrics are not lost on our teenagers — they know exactly what they mean. Other pressures toward premature sexual intercourse are rampant. Illicit sexual relations are pictured not only as fun but as the norm in books, on TV, and in the movies. Provocative sex symbols underlie much of present day advertising. The automobile and rapid mobility allow our youth easily to take advantage of these come-ons.

Many fallacies have emerged concerning premarital sex which mislead young people. Let us look at some of the fallacies and some suggested rebuttals:

"Everybody's doing it; why not go all the way?" Jane asked.

This is an old but flimsy cliché. Even Kinsey, who was in favor of more liberal sexual expression, reported that fifty percent of college males and eighty percent of unmarried women between the ages of sixteen and twenty had had no sexual relations before marriage. Although recent reports show that there is a trend for more and more teenagers to experiment in this way, most indicate that a majority of teenagers are still chaste. So, everybody is not doing it! A lot more people are talking about doing it than really are. Even if everybody were doing it, it is not necessarily right or healthy.

"Since sex urges are normal, shouldn't we have the freedom to express them?"

"There should be free sex as long as no one gets hurt," a freshman college student argued during a bull session. Such arguments for "free sex" have been made by some noted authorities. Kinsey in his report alluded to the fact that the great lovers of the past (Romeo and Juliet, Helen of Troy, etc.) were young teenagers, implying that modern adolescents should have more freedom of sexual expression as these classical lovers did. What he did not mention, however, is that every one of these "great romances" ended in tragedy. Rather than arguing for "sexual freedom," they warn of the dangers of uninhibited sexual expression for young people.

Actually there is no such thing as "free sex." Everything has a price and sex is no exception. Although there are ways to prevent pregnancy and VD, the psychological price is high for premarital sex. In one recent survey on a large college campus, the coital experience of those undergoing psychiatric therapy was four times that of all other girls in the same school. Uncommitted sex is a new name for an old game called "shacking up." The game has always been a disappointment with the female players the big losers. As O. Hobart Mower says in *Reality Therapy*, "The fallacy of eat, drink and be merry for tomorrow we die, is that we usually don't die tomorrow but live to reap the consequences of shortsighted pleasure."

Another common fallacy that traps many teenagers is the "test before you buy" or "test of love" theory. Sometimes girls are presented with the proposition, "If you really love me, prove it." This is a tricky device used by Don Juans since the beginning of time. It is only a device, however. Authoritative studies of sexual behavior of young people show that on the contrary, men are not likely to have premarital relations with girls they love and consider marrying. If they consider a girl a possible candidate for marriage, men are more inclined to protect her and concern themselves with her feelings, desires, and welfare.

Mary had sexual relations with Bob to "prove her love" although she did not really enjoy the experience. One time they had intercourse in the car at the drive-in movie and the other time at his home. Gradually, Bob became much more casual and soon stopped calling her. Mary was left with some bad memories and no place to go.

Most girls who have sexual relations are interested in marriage. Sometimes a boy experiments thinking that he can drop the girl when he is tired of her. Some girls will sense this and deliberately get pregnant, thus trapping the boy into a permanent relationship he did not want. This then becomes an expensive "test of love" that proves nothing but that "emotion is blind."

Another old argument is that premarital sex helps adjustment in marriage. As the argument goes, the more experience one gets, the better he or she will be in bed after marriage. But this is truly a fallacy. The relationship in marriage is much different from the one in premarital sex. Premarital sex is a casual affair for the satisfaction of the "self." Usually it occurs under conditions that are less than ideal. Sexual relationships in marriage are a mutual sharing of oneself with your lover. The chief interest is not yours but your lover's satisfaction. To be a real sexual expert in marriage, one must know the needs and idiosyncrasies of the partner and respond to him or her as a person. Such knowledge or experience does not come from having sexual relationship with many partners before marriage but it comes from loving and living with a person. No amount of technical expertise makes one a good husband or wife.

In the preceding chapters we have emphasized the naturalness of the sex drive experienced by all young people. Some would ask, "Since these sex urges are normal why shouldn't we be allowed to express them?"

The sexual feelings and urges are certainly God-given and are a normal part of human nature. But experience continues to show that for the reasons already mentioned, it is best to postpone full sexual experience until it can be consummated within the bonds of marriage.

Actually such postponement can be healthy. Historian Arnold Toynbee claims that much of the creative energy of the West as we know it today, has come from the postponement of adolescent sexual fulfillment until educational and vocational preparation has been made. Such transfer of sexual energy into creative tasks, called sublimation by Freud, is a powerful drive toward creativity. Permissive cultures have remained at the lowest level of development. The liberal sex morals of the primitives so lauded by Kinsey and others, may be a prime contributor to the fact they are still primitive.

A boy or girl who have a good image of themselves as persons will not have to engage in sexual actions to prove their manhood or womanhood. In fact, those who do seek to prove themselves in this way often have serious doubts about their sexuality.

To the Christian teenager the final answer to "why wait?" is not those already mentioned but this one: God, who created us, commanded that all sexual relationships be saved for marriage. He tells us through the Bible that the full joy and beauty of sexual intercourse can be fully developed within the commitment of marriage. God calls sexual intimacy outside marriage sin, not because He wants to limit our happiness, but on the contrary, He wants us to know the full joy of sex free from guilt. Christ left no room for doubt when he said, "Thou shalt not commit adultery" (Matt. 5:7).

For Christian young people, such waiting can be and often is frustrating. But this frustration is from doing what is right. Engaging in premature sexual intimacies in no way ends the frustration; it only complicates it with new problems and guilt. And the new frustration would be based on doing the wrong thing, not the right.

There is a clear answer to the question "why wait?": Waiting for marriage is the only way a couple can know the true beauty of sex as God intended it to be!

Petting

Handholding, kissing and simply caressing is behavior commonly observed in dating couples who like each other. Such expressions of affection should be limited during early adolescence (as in fact all dating should be limited for this age). However, in high school and college age youth such activities are normal expressions of affection and are harmless when engaged in sparingly. However, when a dating couple get so involved in these activities that they cannot enjoy cultural events and group activities, it is certainly harmful.

Another problem continually faces the dating teenager. How do you stop at simple shows of affection without proceeding into more intense sexual exploration, commonly called necking or petting? The teenager does not always know what to expect of himself or his date or how to keep the situation from getting out of control. Heavy caressing, deep kissing, touching the breasts or genitals produce heightened sexual arousal that drives both sexes toward intercourse. Once aroused, this sexual excitement seeks release.

The teenager is faced with a dilemma. Either he must bring this arousal to an uncomfortable halt or proceed to intercourse. While there is a temptation to be swept away by the emotions of the moment, most teenagers are aware of the dangers of premarital intercourse. The Christian teenager realizes that this violates his personality as well as his body. Thus, it is best for the teenager not to get caught in the spiraling trap of heavy petting.

Parents can help by giving the teenager a positive moral code to live by. As a rule, adolescents are guided by the standards of their family. Parents should keep communications open so that the teen boy or girl will feel free to talk about his or her dilemmas as they arise. Also parents can help by respecting their teen-ager's efforts and avoid suspicion, close questioning, teasing or overly harsh restrictions.

It will also help the maturing teenager to know that his parents had some problems as adolescents and came through them successfully.

Contraception

Contraception is the prevention of pregnancy by various means. It is widely advocated for married couples so that the size and spacing of families can be regulated. This is an important issue today because of the real threat of overpopulation.

There are several methods of contraception.

Rhythm Method: This is called the natural method and is the only one approved by the Catholic Church. It is based on the principle that a woman can get pregnant only during a three or four day period at the time of ovulation, midway through the menstrual cycle. This method simply involves abstaining from sexual intercourse during the period of ovulation. Since the time of ovulation usually cannot be easily predicted, this method is risky.

The Pill: Oral contraceptives consist of hormones that suppress ovulation. If taken as directed, they are ninety-five to hundred percent effective. However, side effects do occur and they should be given only with the supervision of a physician.

Blocking of Sperm in Vagina: This is an old method with many variations. The condom, a rubber balloon worn over the penis is one method. Another is the diaphragm that fits over the neck of the uterus and prevents the entrance of the sperm. The diaphragm has to be inserted each time prior to intercourse. An-other way to accomplish this is through the use of creams, jellies, or foams that kill the sperm in the vagina before they reach the egg. All of these methods are safe but vary in the effectiveness — in general they are not as effective as the pill or IUD.

IUD: The intrauterine device is being used more and more as a means of contraception. The IUD consists of a metal or plastic loop which is inserted into the uterus. It apparently works by preventing the fertilized egg from implanting in the uterus. Some women are not able to use the IUD because of pain or bleeding. But in those who are able to retain it, it is quite effective (almost as good as the pill).

Male Sterilization: This form of contraception is not used too often since it is nearly always permanent. However, it is simple and involves only a minor operation in which the sperm cords are cut as they come near the skin at the base of the scrotum. The surgery can be done in a doctor's office and is quite safe. This technique is sometimes chosen by a husband after his family has reached the desired size.

Some parents and professionals advocate the use of contraceptives on a routine basis by unmarried girls as a means of preventing illegitimate pregnancies. While there is no proof that such a practice increases premarital intercourse, there are reasons why such a plan may not be the best. First of all, some studies have shown that the use of contraceptives by unmarried girls is not entirely effective in preventing illegitimate pregnancies. It seems that the highly emotional teenager is not always capable of using the contraceptives correctly. Also, it is possible that hormones in the oral contraceptives can affect the bone growth in younger adolescent girls. For the Christian parent, the question of single teenagers using contraceptives is a moot one. For the goal of the Christian parent, physician, and teacher is not to just prevent pregnancy, is to help the teenager remain free of the guilt and warped emotions associated with premature sexual intercourse. The ultimate goal is to help them develop a healthy and balanced concept of sex so that they might find fulfillment in marriage.

If after weighing all the factors, your teenagers decide to engage in premarital intercourse whether you approve or not, it would be wise to discuss with them the use of contraceptives. To do so could prevent an even greater evil — an illegitimate pregnancy. However, such a course of action should be taken only after considerable thought and exhaustion of all forms of persuasion, realizing that it is the lesser of two evils.

Abortion

Abortion refers to the termination of a pregnancy by any means before the fetus is mature enough to live outside of the womb.

In general, there are two types of abortions. A spontaneous abortion, commonly called a miscarriage, is the termination of a pregnancy by natural means before the fetus is mature enough to live. Spontaneous abortions have a variety of causes such as a poorly formed egg, illness in the mother, or some abnormality of the womb.

An induced abortion is the termination of a pregnancy by artificial means. Until recently, strict laws regulated the use of induced abortion. It was legally permitted only when necessary to save the life of the mother. In some states the laws now permit induced abortion when the mother's mental or physical health is threatened or when the infant is likely to be severely damaged. Other states have passed laws permitting abortion on demand for any reason.

The question of induced abortion presents a dilemma to the physician. While the life and happiness of the mother must be considered, the life of an unborn person must not be taken lightly. The penetrating question is, "When does an unborn fetus become a person with all the dignity and rights thereof?" Some say that it becomes a person as soon as the egg is fertilized; others would say that it is not a person until it is born.

Thus, the Christian Medical Society's statement on abortion remarks: "The sanctity of life must be considered when the question of abortion is raised. At whatever stage of gestation one considers the developing embryo or fetus to be human, even at birth, the potential great value of the developing intrauterine life cannot be denied. There may, however, be compelling reasons why abortion must be considered under certain circumstances. Each case should be considered individually, taking into account the various factors involved and using Christian principles of ethics."

Homosexuality

Homosexuality, or sexual relations between members of the same sex, is not as uncommon as it was once thought to be. In one study, thirty-seven percent of the men and thirteen percent of the women questioned had homosexual relationships to the point of orgasm, although all of these were not confirmed homosexuals. Four percent of the men and three percent of the women were exclusively homosexual. So it is not an uncommon phenomenon. Today, homosexuals are becoming more visible and vocal.

No consensus exists among authorities as to the cause of homosexuality, but it appears to develop early in life. Some claim that it is inborn and physically determined. There is evidence that homosexuality can be an outgrowth of environmental pressures such as an unsatisfactory social relationship with the opposite sex or prolonged segregation by sex in boarding schools or other institutions. The best evidence, however, indicates that homosexuality develops out of problems of sexual identity in the early years of life. Rejection of the child's sex by his parents, marital unhappiness in his parents, antagonism toward the parent of the opposite sex or strong attraction toward the parent of the same sex all have been pin-pointed as causing homosexuality. Probably there is no one cause but all of these factors work together to influence the child's development of sexual identity.

In previous chapters, it has been pointed out that crises in sexual identity occur at two periods in a child's development. The first is in the first two or three years of life when a child takes the identity of male or female. Chapter 8 discussed the various factors that influence this acquisition of sexual identity. The second crises in sexual identity occurs during early adolescence when both boys and girls often doubt their masculinity or femininity.

Homosexuality does not just suddenly develop in the teenage years. It may become apparent at this time but its roots lie deep in the child's past. Many teenagers in the process of finding their identity, occasionally have homosexual thoughts or fantasies. When concerned about this the teenager can be reassured that such thoughts are normal and one or two such thoughts will not make him or her a "homo."

Stereotyped concepts of what homosexuals look like exist. But contrary to popular belief, there are no appearances that are common to all homosexuals. Sometimes frail, passive men or robust women are unfairly stigmatized as homosexual. Studies have shown that homosexuals cannot be identified by their appearance in this way.

Parents often worry about their children being the victim of a homosexual advance. As a practical matter parents cannot shield their children, particularly boys, from all possibility of such advances. However, if the child has received a healthy concept of sexuality from his parents and if his questions about sex have been answered frankly, the child will likely recoil from the homosexual advance. However, the boy who has been kept in the dark about all things sexual may be unguarded and open to such an advance.

The Bible firmly teaches that homosexuality is a violation of the God-ordained pattern of sexual expression and it is unequivocally prohibited (Rom. 1:27). However, homosexuality like other sins is not unpardonable. Those who practice homosexuality have the same opportunity to receive God's forgiveness as the heterosexual.

Venereal Disease

Venereal diseases are a group of infections acquired by sexual intercourse. The word "venereal" is derived from *Venus*, the Latin Goddess of Love. The bacteria which cause the various venereal diseases live only in human beings and cannot live outside of the body for long. Thus, these diseases are virtually always contracted by means of sexual intercourse.

The most common of the venereal diseases are syphilis and gonorrhea. Both of these are among the most serious medical problems throughout the world and they attack men, women, and children alike. They not only damage the genital organs and cause sterility but may also attack the heart, blood stream, and nervous system.

Since the 1940's, penicillin has been an excellent treatment for both of these diseases. In the 1950's there was optimism about completely eradicating these scourges from the earth. But beginning in the late 1950's, a spiraling increase in the number of VD cases occurred. At the present time, a frightening epidemic of both diseases is spreading over the country and much of the world. Regrettably, teenagers are the group producing most of the new cases. Thus, we have the spectacle of thousands of teenagers, with life ahead of them, risking sterility and chronic disease.

Studies show that there is no typical teenager who is likely to acquire VD. Of young people treated in VD clinics, all personality types are represented. At one time VD was largely a disease of the lower social classes but today it is quite democratic and a significant number of young people from all social classes are represented. Interestingly, twenty-five percent of teenagers treated in a VD clinic were regular attenders at church services. This is just another indication that young people from Christian homes are not shielded from the influence of society and need adequate education to deal with the pressures put on them.

Most revealing is the fact that the teenager with VD is likely to come from a family where there is a lack of communication and wholesome interpersonal relationships. Less than twenty-five percent had received information from their parents on sexual matters. All were ignorant of the basic facts of reproduction biology and hygiene.

VD victims are often young people who see themselves as worthless and unlovable. They seek security and relief of depression through sexual promiscuity. They are encouraged in this by the popular American concept of sex that relates security with love and love with sex. Also in our society, moral and ethical standards are less and less emphasized. Thus, young people have no clear guide to behavior. Unfortunately, VD is often the result. Adolescents who refrain from promiscuous behavior can be assured that they will not become victims of VD. Most teenagers who are presented with the moral and scientific facts will act wisely. Those who are kept in the dark are the ones in danger.

As severe as it is, VD is among the most easily treated diseases if the treatment is started immediately. Thus, if a teenager, or his parent, becomes aware that he has made a mistake and acquired one of the venereal diseases, they should admit the truth quickly and seek medical help. Every day spent in delaying treatment increases the chance of permanent damage. Sooner or later the truth must be faced; the sooner the better.

Questions For Discussion and Thought

1. Can parents really impose sex standards on the older teenager? How can we best assure that our older teenager will act responsibly in sexual situations?

2. What would you do if your son came home from college with his girl friend and declared that they were going to sleep in his room — together?

3. Your sixteen-year-old daughter becomes pregnant. What would you do?

4. Your fifteen-year-old daughter starts dating. Will you tell her about contraceptives? Why or why not? How would you do it?

PART FIVE

◆

When Parents Need Help

Chapter 15

◆

The Church and Sex Education

The Southern Baptist Convention made a survey which showed that young people wanted and needed help in dealing with the personal problems associated with sex. The Convention responded by producing a study series entitled, "Youth Faces Attitudes Toward Sex," which was concerned with Christian answers to current problems of concern to youth. Shortly after the material was made available to the churches, the Sunday School Board received a larger than usual negative response. More than thirty churches returned the materials and letters of opposition were received from individuals, pastors and churches in over eleven states. About the same time a Christian magazine in Texas polled its readers asking whether any form of sex education should be included in the church training program. Those for such a program only barely carried the day with fifty-four percent of those polled for and forty-six percent against. One letter against said, "Why clutter our children's minds? Let them be happy."!!!

Such a negative attitude by many Christian individuals is not only pathetic, but non-Christian. Christ ministered to the whole person — the physical, mental and spiritual nature of the personality. A church that does less is failing in its responsibility to its youth. A church, a pastor, or a Sunday school teacher who does not believe that their young people wish and need help in dealing with sex, is sadly deluded. If Christian young people do not get help from the church, not only they, but the church will suffer.

The youth faced with a church that is silent about sex perceives one of three things:

. . . That the church thinks sex is an unimportant part of life. (The youth cannot believe this because of the intensity of his own feelings.)

. . . That sex or what one does with it has nothing to do with one's relationship to God. (It is hard for the youth to believe that God would be so disinterested in something that so profoundly affects his life.)

. . . That sex must be evil. (This is frequently what young people perceive the church to be saying about sex. All too often, this *is* what the church is saying. Most youth can't believe this either.)

When the church fails to speak up about sex, it loses its young people in spirit, if not in body, and fails to capitalize on one of the most important outreach ministries available today.

What is this valuable ministry available to the church?

In this generation of sexual saturation and emphasis on sexual freedom, young people need, and many want, some authoritative values to hang on to. They need some positive do's and don't's. The church as the representative of God, is qualified to be the anchor in the storm of shifting values of today. If the church will approach young people with honesty about sex, many will listen.

Too often the church has dealt with sex simply by propounding a set of don't's. This will only succeed in turning the young people off. The church can and must present a positive view of sex. While not compromising on standards of sexual conduct, it can show that sex is basically good and God-given. (See Chapters

3 and 4.) The youth need someone who will listen. They do not need a judge, a despotic rule maker, or a policeman.

If the church is silent about sex, young people will turn elsewhere for standards of sexual conduct and sex information. When this happens both the young people and the church are losers.

Some Ideas for a Church Sex Education Program

1. The church and its leaders must first look honestly at their attitudes about sex and see if they truly reflect the biblical view of sexuality. It is the church's responsibility to teach that the Bible sees sex as an important part of life, as a part of life with a positive thrust, and as a part of life that demands responsibility. They need to realize that sexual sins are no greater than sins of lying, cheating, or racial discrimination. Jesus was quick to forgive and accept into His fellowship prostitutes as well as thieves and religious hypocrites.

2. The key to a successful program is openness on the part of the adults working with young people. Many young people do not feel that they can bring their questions and doubts to the leaders and counselors in the church. One teenage boy, a Christian, was shown an article on sexuality in *Playboy* magazine by one of his friends. "I have a lot of the same questions," he said, "But I wouldn't dare discuss them with people at church." How sad! But so true.

3. Teachers and leaders should not be afraid to raise and discuss questions about sex in the regular teaching period of the church. A teacher of a fourteen-year-old boys' Sunday school class was discussing a lesson concerning marriage. He noted that the boys were losing interest and whispering or looking out of the window. He stopped. "Do you ever have sexual feelings?" he

asked. This brought the lesson down to their problems and opened the door for their questions.

"Some of the guys at school say that you don't have to wait until you get married to have sex," one boy responded. "Yea!" another replied. "Did you see the skin flick down at the Martini theater? Whoa, it made me feel funny!"

This teacher listened to the questions and comments of the boys. He had the opportunity to assure them that sexual feelings in themselves were normal and not sinful and that they had no reason to feel guilty. But he also pointed out the dangers and limited rewards of premarital sex and showed how the "skin flick" distorted the true meaning of sex. In the process, he taught the boys more about the biblical material that they were studying than he ever could by following a preplanned talk from the lesson book. He was sensitive to the young people and responded to their needs applying biblical principles to answer their questions.

4. Planned sex education programs for young people are within the capability of many churches. Some ideas for such programs are as follows:

a. Through the use of films or lectures by knowledgeable people such as doctors, nurses, or teachers, a series of programs on physical, emotional, and spiritual aspects of sex can be presented. Many church young people will not pick up the facts at home or at school. As long as the young people are ignorant about the facts, they cannot completely understand the moral aspects of sex. If one had to choose whether his child would learn about the facts of life on the street or at church, I would choose the church because of the atmosphere of reverence and respect that the child would sense from the fact that the church was teaching him these things.

b. A Christian doctor presents a slide program concerning menstruation to a group of preteen girls.

c. An intermediate girls' Sunday school teacher had a series of question and answer sessions where the girls could ask any question they wished about sex.

d. A prepared study series on what the Bible says about sex was taught to one group of young people.

e. Panel discussions with older teenagers on the pro's and con's of abortion, homosexuality, premarital sex, etc., could be arranged.

5. The church can probably make its most successful and long lasting contribution by having an ongoing program of sex education for parents. Many parents have misconceptions about what the Bible says about sex, others are uncomfortable about answering their children's questions and still others are very deficient in knowledge of the facts. If the church can help parents overcome these inhibitions and lack of knowledge, it will contribute greatly to the health and happiness of its children as well as their parents.

The following are some ideas on how the church can establish a sex education program for parents.

a. Have a course in the facts of sex taught by a church physician or nurse at the church.

b. Organize study groups of parents who come together to study methods of dealing with sexual questions of young people and how to answer these questions. These groups can be organized into parents of young children and parents of teenagers for the problems of each group will be somewhat different.

c. This present book can be used in a book study program or in a discussion group of parents.

d. Material on sex education can be included in some of the church's regular training program for adults.

Questions For Discussion and Thought

1. "Why clutter our children's minds? Let them be happy." What is wrong with this attitude toward sex education?

2. From what your church does and does not say, what attitudes about sex does it convey to the youth?

3. What kind of sex education program would you like to see in your church?

4. How would the majority of people in your church react to a sex education program?

Chapter 16

The School and Sex Education

Two places are extremely important in a child's life — his home and his school. Both occupy most of his time during the developing years and he acquires most of his knowledge about life from one or the other of these institutions. This book has emphasized the importance of the home in helping the child acquire proper attitudes toward, and adequate information about, sex.

But is sex education in the home enough? What part can, or should, the school play in teaching children about sex and family life?

Although you may be doing an excellent job of teaching your children about sex and family life, some parents are unable to give their children this information because they don't know how, or don't want to. For their own sake, these children need to be informed about sex and the school is the logical place to do it.

But there is also another compelling reason why all children should be exposed to a proper sex education. For better or worse your children and mine will have to associate with children from a cross section of our society. If their peers and associates are filled with ignorance and myths about sex, our job as parents will be more difficult and our children's confusion will be multiplied. It is also conceivable that one of our children might marry a person from a home where sex education was ignored. In such a circumstance, our child's happiness would be compromised — a fate that could be prevented by proper sex education in the schools.

Thus, most professional people, educators and parents realize that some form of sex education is needed in the schools. In 1930, President Hoover's Conference on Child Health and Protection produced the historic children's charter which set forth nineteen rights of every child. Number eleven states that every child has the right to "teaching and training as will prepare him for successful parenthood, homemaking, and the rights of citizenship."

The 1960 White House Conference on Children and Youth suggested . . . "That the school curriculum include education for family life, including sex education . . . that family life courses, including preparation for marriage and parenthood, be instituted as an integral and major part of public education from elementary school through high school and that this formal education emphasize the primary importance of family life. . . ."

Recently Mary Calderone, head of the Sex Information Council of the United States said that the burden of sex education must be to some extent shouldered by the schools because "of all the institutions of society, the schools are the only ones that have the know-how and the organization and the personnel. Right now it is being romantic and totally unrealistic to say that the child should get all of this kind of education in the home."

Thus, sex education in the schools is needed because the schools are the only institutions that can reach practically all the children over a sustained period of time. Both the easy-to-reach and hard-to-reach are there in the classroom. The latest census reports that from one-fourth to one-third of all children come from broken homes. Often the school is the one stable and authoritative influence in their lives. As an educational institution, the schools are able to pass on the wealth of knowledge about human development, human behavior and family life.

But schools can only do so much. They can complement the efforts of parents and churches. The parents remain the ideal primary source of sex information. The school cannot replace the personal relationship between parent and child or cancel the moral teachings of the church; but a school program can be complementary to these, and alone is better than no sex education at all.

The content, structure of the course, and personnel used in sex education programs in the schools will depend on the local needs and resources. But, in general, the goals of such a program might be as follows:

The Elementary Grades

1. To help each child develop a wholesome attitude toward sex.

2. To ensure the use of the proper terms for all body parts including sex organs.

3. To help children understand the difference between boy and girl.

4. To give direct and correct answers to questions about reproduction.

5. To help each child understand the meaning of the family and how he fits in as a family member.

6. To teach proper techniques of cleanliness.

7. To help preadolescents understand the physical and emotional changes that are and will soon be taking place in their lives.

8. To help young people develop respect for social customs and modes.

These goals can be accomplished in many ways. As with parents, the teacher lays the groundwork for a good sex education by answering honestly any questions the child may ask. A teacher who is not allowed to do this can only confuse the child by evasiveness.

The teacher can answer a child's question frankly, whether it is about Africa or sex, in language that the child can understand. Raising plants and animals in the classroom, visits to farms and zoos and reading stories about family life are some ways that sex education can be introduced in the first, second and third grades.

When the child approaches the fifth and sixth grades more detailed information will be necessary. Boys and girls at these ages feel they have reached a transitional stage in their lives (as indeed they have). They are about to leave the elementary school and move on to the more aggressive intellectual and social demands of junior high. Puberty is advancing, sexual identity is becoming fixed and boy-girl interests are erupting. Formal instruction in plant, animal and human reproduction is appropriate for this age. They are ready to learn about the differences between boys and girls and how babies are made and born. The study of reproduction should follow a logical sequence. Children of this age need to learn that all living things reproduce their own kind. They should acquire an appreciation and wonder of the miracle of creation and reproduction and realize that male and female are necessary for reproduction. They need help in understanding that human mating and reproduction is a responsibility and privilege of marriage.

Goals for Junior and Senior High

1. To give the young person detailed scientific information about mating and reproduction and child care.

2. To help young people develop a reasonable attitude toward sex and relationships with the opposite sex.

3. To present the young person with the facts about venereal disease, premature sexual intercourse, abortion, and premarital pregnancy.

4. To help the young person acquire a background of ideals, standards and attitudes that will guide him or her in choosing a mate.

These goals can be accomplished through formal courses of study, group discussions, panels of professional people, and field work in which the young people work with children in nursery schools, kindergartens, etc. One high school offers a course in family life to boys and girls. They work with prekindergarten children and their parents. Guidance is provided by a high school teacher, a kindergarten teacher, and a parent teacher. Students study such subjects as personality development, human behavior, and family dynamics. Another community has a citizen faculty made up of doctors, nurses, lawyers and clergymen who lead discussions on various questions of interest to the young people. Another school provides for a debate on the pros and cons of such topics as early marriage, premature intercourse, abortion, etc. Such activities provide the young people with the necessary information while at the same time stimulating them to think.

Recently, loud voices have been raised in bitter opposition to sex education. Some of the most vehement and bitter opposition stands under the banner of Christianity although their methods and language often are definitely not Christ-like. Too many crusades against sex education just crusade and do nothing else — they cast such epithets as communism and pornography; they demand that programs be stopped, but they offer no positive alternatives. Those who oppose sex education in the schools play on strong emotions but present few facts. Certainly there are some poor sex education programs in some communities and a poor program may be worse than none at all. But this calls for revision of the program — not abolition. After all, one doesn't stop the teaching of math in school just because the instruction is atrocious. New programs are outlined, appropriate materials acquired, and qualified teachers are trained. The same should be true for sex education.

The real concern of the Christian parent is not whether there should or should not be sex education in the schools; this book has attempted to show the vital necessity of proper sex education. Christian parents should definitely concern themselves with *what kind* of sex education programs the school presents. If they are displeased with the program, apply pressure to modify it, but not to eliminate it. The proper concern of the parent is what is taught and what are the qualifications of the person doing the teaching. As James Huffman said in *Christianity Today,* "The Christian might do well to put his major effort into seeing that sound acceptable courses are developed there rather than into emotional, negative crusades against what are probably inevitable programs."

Having a sex education program in the schools will not be a panacea for all social ills nor will it take the place of the parent as the primary source of information and attitudes. The home will remain the key to the child's understanding of himself and the moral codes by which he is to live.

Questions For Discussion and Thought

1. What are the short-comings of sex education in the public schools?
2. Why is sex education in the schools needed?
3. What kind of people usually oppose sex education? What are their motives?

Glossary

ABDOMEN:

That part of the trunk of the body found between the chest and legs; it contains the stomach, intestines and other organs including the internal sex organs.

ABORTION:

Loss of the fetus from the uterus before it is able to live outside its mother's body, that is before the twenty-sixth to the twenty-eighth week of growth. Abortions are of three types: spontaneous or accidental, criminally induced, and therapeutic. Spontaneous abortion is sometimes referred to as a miscarriage.

ABSTINENCE:

The act of refraining from the use of or indulgence in certain foods, stimulants, or sexual intercourse.

ADOLESCENCE:

The period of life between childhood and adulthood commonly called youth (about age thirteen to twenty for males, about age twelve to nineteen for females); the time when marked physical changes occur in boys and girls, indicating that they are maturing into young men and women.

ADULT:

A fully grown and physically matured man or woman. From the emotional point of view, one who has learned to act responsibly.

ADULTERY:

Sexual intercourse between a married person and an individual other than his or her legal spouse.

AFTERBIRTH:

The placenta and fetal membranes expelled from the uterus following the birth of a child.

AMENORRHEA:

Absence of menstruation.

AMNION:

Thin membrane forming the closed sac or "bag of waters" that surrounds the unborn child within the uterus and contains amniotic fluid in which the fetus is immersed.

AMNIOTIC FLUID:

The fluid in which the fetus is suspended within the amniotic sac.

ANAPHRODISIAC:

A drug or medicine that allays sexual desire.

ANATOMY:

The science of the structure of the body and the relation of its parts.

ANDROGEN:

The male sex hormone.

ANESTHETIC:

An agent or drug which deadens pain.

APHRODISIAC:

Anything, such as a drug or a perfume, that stimulates sexual desire.

AREOLA:

The ring of darkened tissue surrounding the nipple of the breast.

ARTIFICIAL INSEMINATION:

Introduction of male semen into the vagina or womb of a woman by artificial means.

BIRTH:

The process whereby the baby leaves its mother's body and enters the outside world.

BIRTH CANAL:

The passage through which the child is born; includes cervix, vagina and vulva.

BIRTH CONTROL:

Regulation of the birth rate by controlling conception; applied either to the removal of factors which cause conception or to the use of diaphragms, condoms or drugs which prevent ovulation.

BREECH PRESENTATION:

A birth position in which the baby is presented and delivered buttocks first.

CAESAREAN BIRTH (also Caesarean Section):

Delivery of a child through a surgical incision in the abdominal and uterine walls.

CASTRATION:

Removal of the gonads (sex glands) — the testicles in men, the ovaries in women.

CASTRATION COMPLEX:

In psycho-analytic theory, unconscious fears centering around injury or loss of the genitals as punishment for forbidden sexual desires; a male's anxiety about his manhood.

CELIBACY:

The state of being unmarried; abstention from sexual activity.

CERVIX:

The neck of the uterus which expands to permit the baby to enter into the vagina and finally into the outer world.

CHROMOSOME:

A microscopic, rodlike structure found within the cells. Genes, which carry hereditary traits, are located on the chromosomes. Each cell in the body contains forty-six chromosomes, except the sex cells (sperm and ovum) which contain twenty-four chromosomes each.

CIRCUMCISION:

An operation performed on boys (usually when babies) which consists of removing the foreskin or loose flesh that covers the end of the penis.

CLITORIS:

The highly sensitive organ just inside the front and upper end of the vulva, covered by a movable fold of skin, important center of sexual excitement in the female.

COITUS:

Sexual intercourse; the union of the penis and the vagina.

COLOSTRUM:

A thin, milky fluid secreted by the female breasts just before and just after childbirth.

CONCEPTION:

Fertilization of the ovum by the sperm; the moment a woman becomes pregnant due to the union of sperm and ovum within her body.

CONDOM:

A contraceptive used by males consisting of a rubber or gut sheath that is drawn over the erect penis before coitus.

CONGENITAL TRAIT:

A characteristic acquired by an individual before birth but not inherited through the genes; a trait acquired by a child from its mother during pregnancy or birth. For example, a child may be born with a disease contracted from its mother during prenatal life.

CONTRACEPTION:

Prevention of conception.

COORDINATION:

The smooth, harmonious working together of the muscles of the body.

COPULATION:

Sexual intercourse; coitus.

CORD:

The rope-like structure which connects the fetus to the placenta; the umbilical cord.

COURTSHIP:

The events and relationships leading up to, but not necessarily reaching, marriage.

CURETAGE (also Curettement):

Scraping the lining of the uterus with a curette, a spoon shaped medical instrument.

CYTOPLASM:

The jelly-like inner part or living substance of a cell, exclusive of the nucleus; protoplasm.

DOUCHE:

A stream of water or other liquid directed into the vagina for sanitary, medical, or contraceptive reasons.

DYSMENORRHEA:

Painful menstruation.

DYSPAREUNIA:

Coitus that is difficult or painful, especially for a woman.

EGG CELL:

The female sex cell or ovum; when this cell has been penetrated by the male sex cell (sperm), a human embryo is conceived.

EJACULATION:

The discharge of seminal fluid from the penis; an emission.

EMBRYO:

A new life in its earliest stages; in human beings, a "baby" less than three months in prenatal development.

ENDOCRINE:

The system of glands which secretes substances called hormones into the blood stream. Example: pituitary, adrenal and thyroid glands.

ENDOMETRIUM:

The mucous membrane that lines the cavity of the uterus in the female. The nesting place of the embryo.

ERECTION:

The rushing of blood into the penis, causing the tissues to swell and making the penis enlarged and rigid. This condition is a prerequisite to sexual intercourse.

EROGENOUS ZONE:

A sexually sensitive area of the body, such as the mouth, lips, breasts, nipples, buttocks, genitals, or anus.

EROTIC:

Pertaining to sexual arousal or sensation; sexually stimulating.

ESTROGEN:

The female sex hormone.

EUNUCH:

A castrated male.

EXCRETION:

Process of expelling waste from the body.

FALLOPIAN TUBES:

Tubes extending from the uterus to every ovary. The tubes are connected with the uterus, but not directly with the ovaries. They form the passageway for ova from the ovaries to the uterus, and fertilization usually takes place in one of the tubes.

FEMININE:

Like, or of, a woman; having the qualities of a woman; belonging to the female sex.

FERTILE:

Capable of producing or reproducing life. An egg cell is fertile when it has united with a sperm cell. Men and women are fertile when they are able to have children.

FERTILIZATION:

The act or process of becoming fertile; the joining of an egg cell and a sperm cell, producing a human embryo. Fertilization takes place within the mother's body.

FETUS:

A fully developed embryo; an unborn child which usually has been in its mother's uterus at least three months.

FORESKIN:

The cap of skin over the tip of the penis; that which is removed by circumcision; the prepuce.

FORNICATION:

Sexual intercourse between two unmarried people.

FRATERNAL TWINS:

Unlike twins; those who develop from two separate fertilized eggs. They may be of the same or the opposite sex.

FRIGIDITY:

An abnormal aversion to sexual intercourse; the inability of a woman to experience sexual pleasures or gratification during intercourse.

GAMETE:

A sex or reproductive cell of either male or female.

GENE:

A tiny chemical unit which resides on the chromosome and which determines the physical characteristics of the body. Genes carry the family resemblances from the parents to the children.

GENITALS:

The sex organs or reproductive organs, especially those on the outside of the body.

GESTATION:

Pregnancy; the period from conception to birth.

GLAND:

An organ which secretes or excretes chemical substance. The endocrine glands secrete hormones into the blood stream. One of these, the pituitary gland, affects the rate of body growth. There are other glands in the body besides the endocrine glands. The sweat glands, for instance, help to regulate the temperature of the body.

GROWTH:

Multiplication of the cells and development of the body in size, weight, and other features; the process of becoming adult.

GYNECOLOGIST:

A physician who specializes in women's diseases.

GYNECOMASTIA:

Female-like development of the male breasts.

HARLOT:

A lewd woman; a prostitute.

HEREDITY:

The transmission of physical and personality traits from parents to children through the genes of the cells.

HERMAPHRODITE:

An individual possessing both male and female sex glands (ovary and testicle) or sex gland tissue of both sexes.

HETEROSEXUALITY:

Sexual attraction to, or sexual activity with, members of the opposite sex.

HOMOSEXUALITY:

Sexual attraction to, or sexual relations with members of the same sex.

HORMONE:

Any chemical substances formed in the endrocrine glands, which affect the activity or growth of another gland or some part of the body.

HYMEN:

The membrane which covers, or partly covers, the opening of the vagina in most young girls. Its absence does not necessarily prove lack of virginity.

IDENTICAL TWINS:

Twins which develop from a single fertilized ovum which has split in two. They look almost alike and are always of the same sex.

IMPOTENCY:

Sexual inadequacy in the male, corresponding to frigidity in the female.

INCEST:

Sexual relations between close relatives, such as father and daughter, mother and son, or brother and sister.

INHERITED TRAIT:

A characteristic transmitted to a child from its parents by way of the genes; hereditary trait.

LABOR:

The rhythmical muscular movements of the uterus as it forces the baby out of the birth canal in childbearing.

LACTATION:

The secretion of milk from the mother's breasts to feed her baby.

LESBIAN:

A female homosexual.

LIBIDO:

Sexual drive or urge.

MAMMARY GLANDS:

The milk-producing glands located within the breasts of women.

MASCULINE:

Like, or of, a man; having the qualities of a man; belonging to the male sex.

MASTURBATION:

The handling and stimulation of the genital organs in order to receive sexual pleasure.

MATING:

The union of male and female in the reproductive act; the injection of the penis into the vagina, so that the sperm cells can be deposited.

MATURITY:

Adulthood: the state of being fully grown and developed.

MENOPAUSE:

The period of life for women, generally in the middle or late forties, when menstruation ceases.

MENSTRUATION:

A normal shedding of the uterine lining through the vagina, occurring once a month for most women.

MISCARRIAGE:

The loss of the embryo or fetus before it is old enough to live, between the first and sixth month of its growth in the womb. A more proper term is spontaneous abortion.

MOTOR SKILLS:

Ability to control muscles and bodily movements; muscular coordination.

NAVEL:

The place in a person's abdomen where he was joined to the umbilical cord during prenatal life.

NUCLEUS:

The vital center of a cell containing the chromosomes.

NYMPHOMANIA:

Excessive sexual desire in women.

OBSTETRICIAN:

A physician who specializes in taking care of women during pregnancy and who delivers babies.

OVARIES:

The two almond-shaped reproductive glands of the female. They produce egg cells (ova) and certain hormones which have to do with the female's sex functioning and with the development of feminine body characteristics.

OVULATION:

The shedding of eggs from the ovaries; the production of ripe ova.

OVUM:

The female reproductive cell; the egg cell. The egg develops into an embryo when penetrated by a sperm cell.

PEDIATRICIAN:

A physician who specializes in the care of children.

PELVIS:

The structure of bones supporting the trunk of the body and through which a baby must pass at birth.

PENIS:

The male sex organ through which sperm cells leave the body; also used to discharge urine.

"PERIOD":

The several days during each month when a woman menstruates; the menstrual period.

PETTING:

Mutual fondling and caressing.

PHYSIOLOGY:

The study of the constitution and functioning of the body.

PHIMOSIS:

Tightness of the foreskin of the male penis, so that it cannot be drawn back from over the glans.

PIGMENT:

The substance in the body cells which give coloring to the eyes, hair and skin.

PITUITARY:

The small gland which secretes various hormones, including the growth hormone. It is located at the base of the brain.

PLACENTA:

The structure formed in the lining of the uterus during pregnancy to provide for the nourishment of the fetus and for the disposal of its body wastes. It is expelled after delivery, becoming the afterbirth.

PORE:

Tiny opening in the skin through which perspiration passes.

PORNOGRAPHY:

The presentation of sexually arousing material in literature, motion pictures, or other means of communication and expression.

POTENT:

Having the male capability to perform sexual intercourse; capable of erection.

PRECOCIOUS SEXUALITY:

Awakening of sexual desire at a prematurely early age.

PREGNANT:

Condition of a woman expecting a child, a woman with an embryo or fetus in her uterus.

PREMATURE BIRTH:

Birth of a baby before the normal nine-month period has elapsed but after about the twenty-eighth week when the fetus can live outside its mother's body.

PRENATAL:

Referring to the period prior to birth; the period of pregnancy.

PROCREATION:

The process by which a husband and wife reproduce a child through mating; reproduction.

PROMISCUITY:

Indiscriminate immoral relations. Sexual relations with a variety of partners.

PROSTITUTE:

A woman who engages in sexual intercourse for money as a livelihood; a harlot.

PUBERTY:

Sexual maturity or the earliest age at which a person is able to reproduce; occurs at about twelve years of age for girls and at about fourteen years of age for boys. Puberty is marked by certain physical changes, such as the development of the breasts in girls and the growth of the beard for boys.

PUBIC REGION:

That area of the abdomen where the sex organs are found.

RAPE:

Forcible sexual intercourse with a person who does not give consent or who offers resistance.

REPRODUCTION:

The process whereby new individuals are brought to life through the mating of father and mother; procreation.

RHYTHM METHOD:

A method of birth control that relies on the so-called "safe-period" or infertile days in a woman's menstrual cycle.

SCROTUM:

The pouch of skin behind the penis containing the male testes.

SECRETION:

The substance produced by the glands. The secretions of the endocrine glands are called hormones.

SEMEN:

The fluid produced by the testes. It contains sperm cells.

SEMINAL EMISSION:

The discharge of semen from the penis during sleep. It is frequently accompanied by a dream known as a "wet dream."

SEX CELL:

The sperm of the male and the ovum of the female.

SEXUAL INTERCOURSE:

Mating; the uniting of the penis and vagina; coitus, copulation.

SPERM:

The male reproductive cell, which starts a new life by joining with an ovum; spermatozoan.

STERILITY:

The inability to produce offspring.

SUBLIMATION:

The channeling of sexual energies and tensions into nonsexual and approved outlets, such as sports, dramatics, social and charitable activities.

TESTES:

The two male reproductive glands, that manufacture sperm cells and the male sex hormones; testicles. The testes are enclosed in the scrotum.

TRUNK:

The part of the body between the neck and the legs; the chest and abdomen together.

UMBILICAL CORD:

The rope-like structure connecting the embryo or fetus to the placenta. It carries nourishment and oxygen from the mother to the baby.

UNDESCENDED TESTICLE:

A developmental defect in males in which the testicles fail to descend into the scrotum; cryptrochidism.

URINE:

The waste fluids from the kidneys discharged through the penis of the male and through the vulva of the female.

UTERUS:

The chamber where a baby develops before birth, located in the lower part of the woman's abdomen, at the head of the vagina; the womb.

VAGINA:

The passageway from the uterus to the outside of the woman's body; the birth canal; the place where sperm cells are deposited by the penis during mating.

VENEREAL DISEASE:

A disease communicated through sexual intercourse with an infected person.

VERNIX:

The fatty substance covering the skin of the newly born baby.

VIRGIN:

A woman, especially a young woman, who has had no sexual intercourse. May also refer to a young man of the same state.

VULVA:

The two pairs of lips forming the outside part of the female sex organ; the entrance to the vagina.

"WET DREAM":

The discharge of semen from the penis during sleep; a normal function usually accompanied by a dream; noctural or seminal emission.

WOMB:

The uterus; the organ which houses the unborn baby inside its mother.

Supplemental Reading List

The following books serve as additional sources of information about sex for both parents and their children. Some of these are written for parents, others for parents to read to their children, and others are especially for teenagers to read by themselves. This list is not all inclusive but the books selected are representative and for the most part are compatible with the Christian perspective.

FOR PARENTS

Parents' Guide to Christian Conversation About Sex by Erwin J. Kolb. This book is a part of the fine Concordia series on Sex Education. It helps parents answer the child's questions on his level. Concordia Publishing House.

What to Tell Your Child About Sex by the Child Study Association of America. Question and answer style is helpful in dealing with a variety of questions which children ask. This is a handy reference manual in paperback. Child Study Association of America.

Between Parent and Child by Haim Ginott. Delightfully written book which offers practical advice on a variety of child rearing questions including sex education. The Macmillan Company.

Promises to Peter by Charlie Shedd. Written by a popular Christian author and preacher, this book offers valuable insights into parent-child relationships at all levels. Word Books.

Facts Aren't Enough by Marion O. Lerrigo and Helen Southard. This is a seventy-page pamphlet which can be ordered from the American Medical Association (535 North Dearborn Street, Chicago, Ill. 60610) for thirty cents. It contains an adequate, but simple discussion of the physical facts of reproduction.

For Young Children (These books are designed to be read to the child by his parents. Older school children may be able to read some of these books themselves.)

I Wonder, I Wonder by Marguerite Kurth Frey. A delightful story to be read aloud to children five to eight years of age. It is about two small children and a new baby brother. Common questions are answered by means of the story. It gives a very complete explanation. Concordia Publishing House.

Wonderfully Made by Ruth Hummel. Another one of the fine Concordia Series for children ages nine to eleven. Offers a clear presentation of physical and emotional aspects of sexual growth and answers common questions of the age group. Concordia Publishing House.

The Wonderful Story of How You Were Made by Sidonie Gruenberg. Emphasizes the wonder of human birth and reproduction while presenting the appropriate facts.

About Sex and Growing Up by Evelyn Duvall. An excellent comprehensive book for this age group (elementary school age) by a noted expert on sex education. Not only does it deal sensitively with the facts but it does not ignore the moral aspect of sex. Association Press.

For Adolescents

These books are writen primarily for the teenager. However, parents could also benefit from reading them. In some families a warm openness may be established if both parents and teenager read and discuss the books together.

The Stork Is Dead by Charlie Shedd. A very readable book that speaks to the teenager on his own level. It is particularly good for middle to older teens. Its frankness is coupled with a definite Christian perspective.

Love and the Facts of Life by Evelyn Duvall. Well written by one of America's foremost authorities, this book is a classic in its field. It frankly discusses all aspects of sex in a style the teenager can identify with. Association Press.

Why Wait Till Marriage by Evelyn Duvall. Convincingly discusses the reasons for pre-marital chastity. Association Press.

Letters to Karen (for girls) and *Letters to Phillip* (for boys) by Charlie Shedd. These books are made up of letters written by Mr. Shedd to his children at the time of their engagement. Discusses many issues important to young people anticipating marriage including pertinent information about sex in marriage. Abingdon Press (paperback).

Please Help Me, Please Love Me by Walter Trobish. A concise little book consisting of a series of letters between the author and a young African couple. An excellent discussion of the Christian's approach to birth control. (This and several other books by Mr. Trobish are excellent for older teenagers.) Available from Inter-Varsity Press in paperback.

Letters to Chip by Dan Seagren. An imaginary exchange of letters between an older brother and his teen-aged younger brother. Touches on many of the issues and problems of the teen years. Zondervan Publishing House.

Letters to Cindy by Dan Seagren. A similar book reporting the correspondence between an older and younger sister. Sensitive and satisfying. Zondervan Publishing House.

So You're a Teenage Girl by Jill Renich. A mother talks frankly with her teenage daughter and shares insights and information valuable and applicable to all girls. Zondervan Publishing House.

Young Only Once by Clyde M. Narramore. For older teens, deals with many areas of growing up, including the increasing sexual awareness of young people during these years. Zondervan Publishing House.

Sexual Understanding Before Marriage by Herbert J. Miles. A frank discussion of valuable pre-marital counseling subjects. For those young people contemplating marriage. Zondervan Publishing House.

Index

Shame, about sex, 23, 45-46
Sleeping arrangements, 61
Sordid subjects, 113
Song of Songs, 30
Source of sex information, 15
Spitz, Rene, 75
Sunday school, 18, 100, 147, 149
Syphilis, 140

Toilet Training, 81ff

Venereal disease, 17, 140ff

Wet dream, 117
What to teach about sex, 54ff
When to teach about sex, 55ff
White House Conference of Children and Youth, 152